Depression and Cancer

World Psychiatric Association titles on Depression

In recent years, there has been a growing awareness of the multiple interrelationships between depression and various physical diseases. This series of volumes dealing with the comorbidity of depression with diabetes, heart disease and cancer provides an update of currently available evidence on these interrelationships.

Depression and Diabetes
Edited by Wayne Katon, Mario Maj and Norman Sartorius
ISBN: 9780470688380

Depression and Heart Disease
Edited by Alexander Glassman, Mario Maj and Norman Sartorius
ISBN: 9780470710579

Depression and Cancer
Edited by David W. Kissane, Mario Maj and Norman Sartorius
ISBN: 9780470689660

Related WPA title on depression:

Depressive Disorders, 3e
Edited by Helen Herrman, Mario Maj and Norman Sartorius
ISBN: 9780470987209

For all other WPA titles published by John Wiley & Sons Ltd, please visit the following website pages:

http://eu.wiley.com/WileyCDA/Section/id-305609.html

http://eu.wiley.com/WileyCDA/Section/id-303180.html

Depression and Cancer

Editors

David W. Kissane
*Department of Psychiatry and Behavioral Sciences, Memorial
Sloan-Kettering Cancer Center, New York, NY, USA*

Mario Maj
*Department of Psychiatry, University of Naples SUN,
Naples, Italy*

Norman Sartorius
*Association for the Improvement of Mental Health
Programmes, Geneva, Switzerland*

WILEY-BLACKWELL

A John Wiley & Sons, Ltd., Publication

This edition first published 2011 © 2011, John Wiley & Sons, Ltd.

Wiley-Blackwell is an imprint of John Wiley & Sons, formed by the merger of Wiley's global Scientific, Technical and Medical business with Blackwell Publishing.

Registered office: John Wiley & Sons Ltd, The Atrium, Southern Gate, Chichester, West Sussex, PO19 8SQ, UK

Editorial Offices: 9600 Garsington Road, Oxford, OX4 2DQ, UK
           The Atrium, Southern Gate, Chichester, West Sussex, PO19 8SQ, UK
           111 River Street, Hoboken, NJ 07030-5774, USA

For details of our global editorial offices, for customer services and for information about how to apply for permission to reuse the copyright material in this book please see our website at www.wiley.com/wiley-blackwell

Library of Congress Cataloguing-in-Publication Data

Depression and cancer / editors, David W. Kissane, Mario Maj, Norman Sartorius.
     p. ; cm.
     Includes bibliographical references and index.
     ISBN 978-0-470-68966-0 (pbk.)
  1. Cancer–Psychological aspects. 2. Depression, Mental. I. Kissane, David W. (David William)
II. Maj, Mario, 1953– III. Sartorius, N.
    [DNLM: 1. Depressive Disorder–etiology. 2. Neoplasms–complications. 3. Neoplasms–psychology. WM 171]
    RC262.D47 2011
    616.99′40019—dc22

                          2010029174

A catalogue record for this book is available from the British Library.

This book is published in the following electronic formats: ePDF 9780470972526; Wiley Online Library 9780470972533

Set in 10/12 Pt Times by Thomson Digital, Noida, India.
Printed and bound in Singapore by Fabulous Printers Pte Ltd

First Impression   2011

Contents

List of Contributors

William Breitbart   Department of Psychiatry and Behavioral Sciences, Memorial Sloan-Kettering Cancer Center, New York, NY, USA

David M. Clarke   School of Psychology and Psychiatry, Monash University, Melbourne, VIC, Australia

M. Robin DiMatteo   Department of Psychology, University of California, Riverside, CA, USA and Texas State University, San Marcos, TX, USA

Pernille Envold Bidstrup   Department of Psychosocial Cancer Research, Danish Institute of Cancer Epidemiology, Danish Cancer Society, Copenhagen, Denmark

Luigi Grassi   Section of Psychiatry, Department of Medical Sciences of Communication and Behaviour, University of Ferrara, Italy

Sarah Hales   Department of Psychosocial Oncology and Palliative Care, Princess Margaret Hospital, Toronto, ON, Canada

Kelly B. Haskard-Zolnierek   Department of Psychology, University of California, Riverside, CA, USA and Texas State University, San Marcos, TX, USA

Greg Irving   Academic Palliative and Supportive Care Studies Group (APSCSG), School of Population, Community and Behavioural Sciences, University of Liverpool, UK

Christoffer Johansen   Department of Psychosocial Cancer Research, Danish Institute of Cancer Epidemiology, Danish Cancer Society, Copenhagen, Denmark

David W. Kissane   Department of Psychiatry and Behavioral Sciences, Memorial Sloan-Kettering Cancer Center, New York, NY, USA

Elissa Kolva   Department of Psychiatry and Behavioral Sciences, Memorial Sloan-Kettering Cancer Center, New York, NY, USA

Tomer Levin   Department of Psychiatry and Behavioral Sciences, Memorial Sloan-Kettering Cancer Center, New York, NY, USA

Mari Lloyd-Williams   Academic Palliative and Supportive Care Studies Group (APSCSG), School of Population, Community and Behavioural Sciences, University of Liverpool, UK

Christopher Lo   Department of Psychosocial Oncology and Palliative Care, Princess Margaret Hospital, Toronto, ON, Canada

Amy E. Lowery   Department of Psychiatry and Behavioral Sciences, Memorial Sloan-Kettering Cancer Center, New York, NY, USA

Mary Jane Massie   Department of Psychiatry and Behavioral Sciences, Memorial Sloan-Kettering Cancer Center, New York, NY, USA

Marcia D. McNutt   Laboratory of Neuropsychopharmacology, Department of Psychiatry and Behavioral Sciences, Emory University School of Medicine, Atlanta, GA, USA

Andrew H. Miller   Laboratory of Neuropsychopharmacology, Department of Psychiatry and Behavioral Sciences, Emory University School of Medicine, Atlanta, GA, USA

Kimberley Miller   Princess Margaret Hospital, Toronto, ON, Canada

Dominique L. Musselman   Laboratory of Neuropsychopharmacology, Department of Psychiatry and Behavioral Sciences, Emory University School of Medicine, Atlanta, GA, USA

Maria Giulia Nanni   Section of Psychiatry, Department of Medical Sciences of Communication and Behaviour, University of Ferrara, Italy

Susanne Oksbjerg Dalton   Department of Psychosocial Cancer Research, Danish Institute of Cancer Epidemiology, Danish Cancer Society, Copenhagen, Denmark

Steven D. Passik   Department of Psychiatry and Behavioral Sciences, Memorial Sloan-Kettering Cancer Center, New York, NY, USA

Hayley Pessin   Department of Psychiatry and Behavioral Sciences, Memorial Sloan-Kettering Cancer Center, New York, NY, USA

Michelle Riba   Department of Psychiatry, University of Michigan, Ann Arbor, MI, USA

Gary Rodin   Department of Psychosocial Oncology and Palliative Care, Princess Margaret Hospital, Toronto, ON, Canada

Erica B. Royster   Laboratory of Neuropsychopharmacology, Department of Psychiatry and Behavioral Sciences, Emory University School of Medicine, Atlanta, GA, USA

Yosuke Uchitomi   Department of Neuropsychiatry, Okayama University, Okayama, Japan

Preface

Cancer affects close to one in two men and women across their lifetime, with this risk increasing steadily with age. In many countries, cancer competes with heart disease to become the leading cause of death, while being arguably the major cause of health morbidity, given the many losses, including disfigurement, disability and impairment, associated with the disease and its treatment. Psychological reactions to these losses are many, ranging from demoralization and passivity to anger and memory problems. In addition, depressive disorders are often comorbid with cancer. The likelihood of general practitioners and oncologists seeing patients with depression in the context of their care for people with cancer is extremely high.

The diagnosis of cancer is perceived by many to be their death sentence. The related existential threat initiates substantial suffering, all the more so if pain is persistent, hopes are dashed, fears fueled, grief intensified and the person feels alone. Such suffering results in much dismay and despair. Whatever the therapy – surgery, radiation, chemotherapy, hormones, vaccines or targeted molecular treatments – the burden of the immediate, long-term and late effects of these regimens adds to the inherent distress. Metaphors of waging war and battlefields fortify against the images of an insidious and uncontrollable spread of disease. In some societies, the word 'cancer' remains unspeakable; for others, its prognosis is never acknowledged. The psychological hurdles to adaptation are formidable.

While its diagnosis readily precipitates a mid-life crisis, cancer recurrence induces deep angst as the prospect of cure fades. The very meaning of existence may be called into question. Worldwide, cancer accounts for nearly 14 per cent of all deaths, but this rises to 25 per cent in Western societies. No family escapes its experience. The treatment of metastatic cancer models the journey of a chronic medical illness for diseases like breast cancer, whereas for others, like pancreatic malignancy, the focus is essentially palliative and on quality of life. The challenge of holistic care has spawned the birth of a new discipline, named *psycho-oncology*, drawing its practitioners from psychiatry, psychology, social work and a range of related mental healthcare providers to deliver psychosocial care to cancer patients and their families. In many countries, they work alongside hospice and palliative care practitioners in providing care during the end-of-life; in others, they reach into genetic counseling services, transplant programs, smoking cessation clinics, cancer prevention and screening units, and, of course, cancer survivorship programs. Consultation-liaison psychiatry services almost always have key involvement with oncology and palliative care programs. For all of these psycho-oncology services, the treatment of cancer patients who develop depressive disorders becomes the bedrock of care.

Currently, the USA estimates that over 12 million cancer survivors exist in its society. New hurdles to adjustment are recognized as these patients transition into survivorship. For some, this is the first time that the busyness of a therapeutic schedule eases and the chance to accept their new reality emerges. For others, coping with the morbidity of their treatment challenges their body image, self-worth, sexuality, fertility, fitness or functionality. Whether living with an amputated limb, lymphedema necessitating daily arm compression, xerostomia only ameliorated by the constant sipping of water, or the need for multiple reconstructive surgeries to sustain cosmesis, the rehabilitative challenges after primary cancer treatment are substantial. As we reflect on the life-cycle of the cancer journey, its cumulative experience of grief, transition and loss, the many challenges to optimal adaptation and quality of life become apparent.

Against this background of the ubiquitous burden of a malignant diagnosis and its treatment, this book focuses upon the relationship between cancer and depression. Major human suffering results from this association, suffering that we can effectively assuage. We begin with an appraisal of its prevalence by Mary Jane Massie and colleagues to make explicit the size of this problem. With cancer's additional dimension of existential threat, both major and subthreshold depressive states enlarge this burden of illness, bringing clinical challenges of definition and recognition to the fore.

The subjective experience of depression in oncology patients results from the interplay of complex gene-environment interactions, involving the biology of the brain with the biology of the cancer and the adaptation of the person. Not only does cancer and its treatment interact often with the hypothalamic-pituitary-adrenal system, but cancers also produce a variety of circulating proteins or cytokines that cross the blood-brain barrier and interact with the mood regulating circuits of the limbic system. Dominique Musselman and her research colleagues elucidate the contribution of these cytokine cascades. A detailed chapter on the pharmacologic treatment of depression by Luigi Grassi and colleagues pays careful attention to the potential for drug-drug interactions, which arise frequently in cancer care.

The psychosocial challenges of cancer to each person's coping necessitates adaptation through grief and mourning, coming to terms with loss and change, and then moving forward with life. Whenever depression interferes with these processes, its form can span sub-threshold to clinical presentations. Furthermore, the existential realm adds death anxiety, aloneness, loss of meaning and control to this equation, bringing states of demoralization into tension with depression. David Clarke focuses on this in a chapter on psychological adaptation to cancer, while later David Kissane, Gary Rodin and colleagues present the broad range of psychotherapeutic modalities that can be added to our pharmacologic armamentarium to improve outcomes.

Screening to increase recognition of depression has proven necessary in oncological care because of the unfortunate tendency for clinicians from every discipline to blur the sadness of the predicament with the prevailing mental health reality. Steven Passik covers the range of available measures to screen for depression and the service issues associated with their clinical application.

William Breitbart and colleagues describe the increased rate of suicide among cancer patients in their chapter on the desire for hastened death. Requests for physician-assisted suicide can be a cry for help and clinicians need considerable experience to tease out the many confounding influences that predispose to, precipitate and perpetuate affective disorders.

Depression is a recognised risk factor for shortened survival from cancer, this outcome being partly mediated through patients' adherence to anti-cancer treatments. Unrecognized depression could bring increased morbidity to bear through this mechanism. Meta-analyses by Robin DiMatteo and Kelly Haskard-Zolnierek about the impact of depression on treatment compliance in medical illness make explicit the inherent issues here.

Finally, the social cost of depression is pronounced, and this burden is felt as much in cancer care as with other medical illness. The roles of culture and socioeconomic status are pertinent. Noteworthy social disparities exist in cancer survival. The health beliefs occurring in African Americans, Asians, Hispanics or Europeans affect cancer outcomes, as does their socioeconomic status. Irrespective of access to cancer care, including in Scandinavian societies where health insurance is universal, those living in poor socioeconomic circumstances die earlier. Using Denmark's national medical record system, Christoffer Johansen and colleagues conclude our book by providing methodologically sound evidence that stress, depression, personality and major life events do not cause the onset of cancer. However, untreated depression and social disparity impact cancer survival, making the treatment of affective disorders a paramount public health concern for every society.

This volume on depression and cancer is part of a WPA series on the comorbidity of mood disorders with various medical illnesses, including heart disease and diabetes. We are grateful to our authors who have given generously of their time and scholarship, to our publishers at Wiley-Blackwell, and to the WPA, through which we hope that the care of depressed patients will steadily improve. Cancer brings a huge social burden; untreated depression adds enormously to any suffering; we have many tools to ameliorate this and improve patients' wellbeing. Let us help those who become weary of life to renew its vigour and joy, with appreciation for life's value, meaning and purpose, despite the diagnosis of cancer.

David W. Kissane
Mario Maj
Norman Sartorius

CHAPTER 1

The Prevalence of Depression in People with Cancer

Mary Jane Massie
Department of Psychiatry and Behavioral Sciences,
Memorial Sloan-Kettering Cancer Center,
New York, NY, USA

Mari Lloyd-Williams and Greg Irving
Academic Palliative and Supportive Care Studies Group (APSCSG),
School of Population, Community and Behavioural Sciences,
University of Liverpool, UK

Kimberley Miller
Princess Margaret Hospital, Toronto, ON, Canada

Depression is amongst the main causes of disability worldwide, leading to personal suffering and increased mortality. The US National Comorbidity Survey revealed a 12-month prevalence of major depressive disorder of 6%, with a lifetime prevalence of 16%, while high comorbidity exists with anxiety disorders, substance use disorders and impulse control disorders [1]. In any twelve-month period, more than half the patients with major depressive disorder are diagnosed with an additional anxiety disorder. Patients with comorbid

Depression and Cancer   Edited by David W. Kissane, Mario Maj and Norman Sartorius
© 2011 John Wiley & Sons, Ltd

depression and anxiety disorders experience more severe symptoms, have a longer time to recovery, use more healthcare resources and have poorer outcome than do those with a single disorder [2]. Seedat *et al.* [3] found that, across cohorts from 15 countries, women developed depression almost twice as frequently as men.

When comorbid with medical illness, depression increases the symptom burden and functional impairment, and worsens medical outcomes [4]. Early studies of depression in the medically ill used patient self-report and varied measures, with a heterogeneous mix of hospitalized medical and surgical patients, and reported prevalence rates ranging from 20 to 30% [5]. In 1987, a retrospective review of 263 000 patients from 327 hospitals found that 24% of those receiving a psychiatric consultation were depressed [6]. However, Snyder *et al.* [7], using both clinical interview and DSM-III-R criteria reported less depression (6%), but more adjustment disorder with depressed mood (14%), in 944 medically ill patients referred for psychiatric consultation.

Wells *et al.* [8] examined Epidemiological Catchment Area Study data regarding mental disorders amongst persons with at least one of eight chronic medical conditions. Six-month and lifetime prevalence rates of mental disorders were increased in those with versus without medical illness (25 and 42% versus 17 and 33%). Thirteen per cent of the chronically medically ill had a lifetime diagnosis of affective disorder versus 8% of those free from medical illness.

Lifetime rates of depression in patients with neurological conditions range from 30 to 50% [9]. Prevalence rates of depression in patients with other medical or systemic illnesses show a variable picture, with the highest rates observed with endocrine disturbances such as Cushing's disease and surprisingly low rates documented in end-stage renal disease.

PREVALENCE OF DEPRESSION IN CANCER PATIENTS

Using DSM-III criteria through a structured clinical interview, the Psychosocial Collaborative Oncology Group (PSYCOG) was one of the first groups to carefully determine the prevalence of mental disorders in 215 randomly selected hospitalized and ambulatory adult cancer patients in three cancer centres [10]. Forty-seven per cent of the patients evaluated had clinically apparently psychiatric disorders. Of these patients, over two-thirds (68%) had adjustment disorders with depressed or anxious mood, 13% had a major depression, 8% had an organic mental disorder, 7% had a personality disorder, and 4% had a preexisting anxiety disorder. The authors concluded that nearly 90% of the mental disorders observed were reactions to or manifestations of disease or treatment. Personality and anxiety disorders can complicate cancer treatment, and were described as antecedent to the cancer diagnosis. This epidemiologically sound study has remained the gold standard for many years.

Many research groups have assessed depression in cancer patients along the years [10–69], and the reported prevalence varies quite widely (major depression 3 to 38%; depression spectrum syndromes 1.5 to 52%). The following databases were searched to retrieve references published between 1965 and 2009: PubMed, Embase, CINAHL (nursing), PsycINFO, Scopus, Science Citation Index/Social Sciences Citation Index, Cochrane Evidence Based Medicine database. The searches were limited to English language references and to studies with more than 100 subjects, where this information was indicated. Table 1.1 shows the 60 studies with more than 100 patients that provided information about the number of patients interviewed and cancer type(s), evaluation methods, and per cent with depression or affective syndromes. Most authors reported patient gender and hospitalization status. The reported prevalence varies significantly because of varying conceptualizations of depression, different criteria used to define depression, differences in methodological approaches to the measurement of depression, and different populations studied.

In early, typically cross-sectional studies, the rate of depression was usually reported for adults with mixed types and stages of cancer. Depression was reported by severity (borderline, mild, moderate, severe, and extreme), or by a symptom such as depressed mood, or by some of these diagnostic categories: major depression, minor depression, depressive disorder, adjustment disorder with depressed mood, or dysthymia, limiting our ability to compare studies. Although many research groups reported the gender and age (usually older) of study subjects, findings usually were not reported by demographic variables, and racial minorities were always underrepresented.

Table 1.1 Representative studies of the prevalence of depression in cancer patients (adapted from Massie [5])

Study	N	Patients	Method	Percent depressed	Specific findings
Fras et al. [11]	110	Pancreatic and colon cancer	Semi-structured interview; MMPI	50% (pancreas); 13% (colon)	76% psychiatric symptoms in those with pancreatic cancer; psychiatric symptoms appeared before other symptoms in patients with pancreatic cancer
Morris et al. [12]	160	Breast biopsy and mastectomy patients; British cohort	Interview; HRSD	22% depression in mastectomy	Mastectomy patients had persistent depression (22%) at 2 yr compared to benign biopsy patients (8%)
Maguire et al. [13]	201	117 ambulatory breast cancer patients; 89 benign disease; British cohort	Clinical interview	26% moderate or severe depression after mastectomy	Control benign patients had 12% depression
Silberfarb et al. [14]	146	Hospitalization status not indicated; 34% primary disease; 36% recurrent; 30% advanced, all breast cancer; US cohort	Structured interview; open-ended questions; modified psychiatric status scale	10% depression in primary cancer diagnosis; 15% in recurrent; 4.5% in advanced cancer	Physical disability did not relate to emotional disturbances; first recurrence of breast cancer most disturbing time; advanced patients had the least depression

Study	N	Sample	Method	Results	Comments
Derogatis et al. [10]	215	Half hospitalized, half ambulatory; all sites and all stages, randomly selected; US cohort	DSM-III criteria; SCL-90; RDS; GAIS; Karnofsky Rating Scale	6% major depression 12% adjustment disorder with depressed mood; 13% adjustment disorder with mixed emotional features	Excluded severely ill (Karnofsky < 50); 47% received DSM-III diagnosis; 68% of these diagnoses were adjustment disorder
Farber et al. [15]	141	Ambulatory; primarily breast cancer	SCL-90	19% severe; 21% moderate; 14% mild	A comparison of males and females with clinical and global scales of the SCL-90 showed no significant differences
Hughes [16]	134	Lung cancer	Structured clinical interview	16% depressed	Most of the depressed patients were depressed before physical symptoms began
Lansky et al. [17]	500	85% ambulatory; 43% survivors with no evidence of disease; 34% early stage	DSM-III, organic brain syndrome section of the PDI; HRSD, Zung SDS; visual pain analogue line	5.3% (using HRSD and SDS); 4.5% (using DSM-III criteria)	
Holland et al. [18]	218	Ambulatory; 107 advanced pancreatic, 111 advanced gastric; US cohort	POMS	21 median POMS gastric; 38 median POMS pancreatic scores	Pancreatic cancer patients had higher depression than gastric cancer amongst men only
Devlen et al. [19]	120	Ambulatory; Hodgkin's disease and non-Hodgkin's lymphoma	Semi-structured interview	8% depressed in year after treatment	Prospective study with interviews at baseline, 2, 6, and 12 mo after diagnosis

(continued)

Table 1.1 (*Continued*)

Study	N	Patients	Method	Percent depressed	Specific findings
Lasry et al. [20]	123	Hospitalized breast cancer	CES-D	50% mastectomy; 50% lumpectomy with radiation; 41% lumpectomy	Depression varied with treatment
Stefanek et al. [21]	126	Ambulatory; mixed; US cohort	BSI	33% depressed; 9% severe; 24% moderate	20% high psychiatric distress in general
Pettingale et al. [22]	168	Hospitalized early breast cancer and lymphoma; all stages; British cohort	Interview; STAI; Wakefield	Major depression not cited	In lymphoma patients, the more advanced the disease, the higher the depression. No correlation with disease state and depression in breast cancer
Grassi et al. [23]	196	Hospitalized and ambulatory; recent diagnosis of cancer; mixed, 18–70 yr; Italian cohort	HRSD; IBQ; interview	24–38% depressed depending on threshold used	38% depression with HRSD cutoff of 17; 24% with HRSD of 21
Hardman et al. [24]	126	Hospitalized; mixed; British cohort	Structured interview GHQ	3% pure depression; 23% mixed anxiety and depression	Psychiatric symptoms related to feeling moderately or severely ill and previous psychiatric illness, but not with awareness of having cancer

Study	N	Population	Assessment	Prevalence	Findings
Fallowfield et al. [25]	269	Stage I and II breast cancer assessed 2 wk, 3 mo, 12 mo after surgery; British cohort	Interview	21% mastectomy; 19% lumpectomy	Less depression in mastectomy and lumpectomy patients given treatment choice
Kathol et al. [26]	152	Mixed; US cohort	DSM-III and DSM-III-R criteria; RDC; Endicott substitution criteria; HRSD; BDI	25–38% major depression, depending on diagnostic system; 19% (depressive symptoms)	Authors concluded that self- and observer-rated scales are sufficient to screen at risk patients but not to diagnose
Colon et al. [27]	100	Hospitalized acute leukaemia; US cohort	DSM-III-R criteria	1% major depression; 2% organic affective syndrome; 8% adjustment disorder	Illness status, depressed mood and perceived social support independently affected outcome; depressed patients had poorer outcome
Hopwood et al. [28]	222	Ambulatory; advanced breast cancer; British cohort	HADS; RSCL	9% depression and 9% anxiety using HADS; 22% affective disorder using RSCL	HADS and RSCL detected different groups of cases; one third of depressed patients persisted for 1–3 mo

(continued)

Table 1.1 (*Continued*)

Study	N	Patients	Method	Percent depressed	Specific findings
Goldberg et al. [29]	320	Newly diagnosed, hospitalized for breast cancer surgery	Modified RSCL; pre-operative, 6 and 12 mo post-operatively	32% depressed malignant; 24% depressed benign biopsy	At 1 yr depression had decreased (21% depressed) in both groups
Maraste et al. [30]	133	Ambulatory; adjuvant radiotherapy; breast cancer	HADS	1.5% depressed; 14% anxiety	Age and surgery-related anxiety; anxiety in ages 50–59 was 44% in mastectomy vs. 4% in conservative surgery
Sneed et al. [31]	133	Hospitalized; newly diagnosed; mixed sites and stages	BSI; HIS-GWB	Major depression not cited	Women with gynaecological and breast cancer had less depression, anxiety, hostility, somatization, psychological distress than men and women with other cancers
Carroll et al. [32]	809	Various cancer sites; US cohort	HADS	17.7% anxiety disorder 9.9% depressive disorder	
Cathcart et al. [33]	257	Ambulatory; women with node negative breast cancer; 155 women received tamoxifen; 102 received no tamoxifen	Clinical interview	15% in tamoxifen treated group; 3% in those not receiving tamoxifen	4.5% of 155 women receiving tamoxifen had to discontinue it secondary to depression

Study	N	Population	Instruments	Results	Comments
Pinder et al. [34]	139	86 hospitalized, 53 ambulatory advanced breast cancer; British cohort	HADS interview	13% depressed; 25% anxiety or depression	Depression more prevalent in low socioeconomic class, in poor performance states, and closer proximity to death
Sneeuw et al. [35]	556	Ambulatory stage I and II breast cancer; interviewed at least 1.5 yr after treatment	DSM-III criteria; DIS; CES-D; SCL-25	4.5% depressed; 6.3% generalized anxiety disorder; 8.8% phobic disorder	Depressive symptoms at one and a half years after treatment and longer; no significant differences in patients who had mastectomy vs. conservative treatment
Kelsen et al. [36]	130	Pancreatic cancer; US cohort	BDI; BHS; MPAC; FLIC	38% depressed (scores $\geq$ 15 BDI)	
Aass et al. [37]	716	Various cancer sites; Norwegian cohort	HADS, EORTC QLQ033, HOC Questionnaire	9% depression; 15% anxiety	
Berard et al. [38]	456	Breast; head and neck; lymphoma	HADS; BDI; Structured psychiatric Interview	14% depression overall; 8% depression (overlap with both scales)	
Kissane et al. [39]	303	Early stage breast cancer; Australian cohort	MILP; HADS; EORTC-QLQ	45% DSM psychiatric disorder; 42% depression and/or anxiety; 27.1% minor depression; 9.6% major depression	8.6% DSM anxiety disorder

(continued)

Table 1.1 (*Continued*)

Study	N	Patients	Method	Percent depressed	Specific findings
Montazeri et al. [40]	129	Lung cancer; Scottish cohort	HADS (administered at baseline and follow-up); QLQ	*Baseline*: 6% borderline anxiety; 10% severe anxiety; 11% borderline depression; 12% severe depression *Follow-up*: 11% borderline anxiety; 10% severe anxiety; 22% borderline depression; 32% severe depression	
Hammerlid et al. [41]	357	Head and neck cancer; Swedish & Norwegian cohort	HADS (administered at 6 different times)	19%–71% probable anxiety; 18%–51% probable depression	
Bodurka-Bevers et al. [42]	246	Epithelial ovarian cancer	CES-D; state anxiety sub-scale of STAI; QOL	21% CES-D depression; 29% anxiety	
Chen et al. [43]	203	Solid and liquid tumours; Taiwanese cohort	HADS	12% anxiety; 20% depression	
DeLeeuw et al. [44]	197	Head and neck cancer	Social Provisions Scale; CES-D; EORTC QOL C30 + 3	29% possible depression (before treatment); 28% possible depression (after 6 mo)	

Study	N	Sample	Assessment	Findings	Comments
Hopwood et al. [45]	987	526 small cell lung cancer; 461 non-small cell lung cancer; British cohort	HADS, Quality of Life Form	33% depression, self-reported; 21% depression and anxiety	Higher prevalence for small cell lung cancer patients
Kugaya et al. [46]	107	Head and neck cancer; newly diagnosed; Japanese cohort	Clinical interview with DSM-III; SCID; HADS	13.1% adjustment disorder 3.7% major depression 15.9% past history of major depression 33.6% alcohol dependence	6.5% alcohol abuse 32.7% nicotine dependence
Pascoe et al. [47]	504	Various cancer sites; Australian cohort	HADS	11.5% anxiety 7.1% depression	
Skarstein et al. [48]	568	Various cancer sites; European	HADS; EORTC QLQC33	9% depression, 13% anxious, 17% psychiatric distress, 5% depression and anxiety	HADS more accurate for depression; EORTC-QLQ good for anxiety, but underdiagnosed depression
Akechi et al. [49]	148	Post operative ambulatory breast cancer; Japanese cohort	HADS	23% psychiatric morbidity; 5% depression	
Akechi et al. [50]	129	Non-small cell lung cancer; Japanese cohort	Clinical Interview, DSM-III	4.7% major depression; 13.9% adjustment disorders	

(continued)

Table 1.1 (*Continued*)

Study	N	Patients	Method	Percent depressed	Specific findings
Ciaramella *et al.* [51]	100	Various cancer sites	Interview; SCID; Endicott HAMD	49% all DSM depressive disorders with SCID; 29% depression with Endicott;	28% depression with both diagnostic criteria
DeLeeuw *et al.* [52]	197 initially; 123 at the end of 3 yr	Head and neck cancer	CES-D; EORTC QQL C30 + 3	42% depression between 6 mo and 3 yr after treatment	
Sharpe *et al.* [53]	3938 screened 570 interviewed	Various cancer sites; breast cancer over-represented; UK cohort	HADS – all patients SCID for HADS high scorers	23% 15 or more on HADS; 34% of HADS high scorers had major depression	8% of entire sample had major depression
Atesci *et al.* [54]	117	Various cancer sites	SCID, HADS, GHQ	13.7% major depression	
Kissane *et al.* [55]	503	Breast cancer (303 early stage; 200 advanced); Australian cohort	MILP, HADS	37% DSM depressed (major depression, dysthymia, adjustment disorder) early stage; 31% advanced disease	Early stage: 9.6% major depression, 27.1% minor depression; Metastatic: 6.5% major depression, 24.5% minor depression
Nan *et al.* [56]	108	Mixed digestive tract cancers	Zung SDS	50% SDS index > 50	

Litofsky et al. [57]	598	High-grade gliomas	SF-36 Mental Health scores	93% patient-reported depressive symptoms; 15% physician-reported depression in postoperative period;	Patient-reported depressive symptoms persisted at 3 and 6 mo; physician-reported depression increased to 22% at 3 and 6 mo
Thomas et al. [58]	236	Various cancer sites; Indian cohort	HADS	20% depressed (8% definite cases)	
Montazeri et al. [59]	177	Breast cancer	HADS	29% severe depression	
Wedding et al. [60]	213	Various cancer sites	BDI	8% major depression; 19% mild to moderate depressive symptoms	
Steel et al. [61]	101	Hepatobiliary	CES-D	37% at diagnosis	
Lueboontha-vatchai. [62]	300	Breast cancer; Thai cohort	Thai HADS	9% depressive disorder; 16.7% depressive symptoms	
Arnold et al. [63]	363	Primary brain tumours	Modified Brief PHQ	41% depression 48% generalized anxiety disorder	
Wedding et al. [64]	175	Various cancer sites	BDI	16.6% mild to moderate depression; 9.1% major depression	

(continued)

Table 1.1 (*Continued*)

Study	N	Patients	Method	Percent depressed	Specific findings
Singer et al. [65]	250	Laryngeal cancer	HADS	9.7% depressed; 5.2% major depression, 4.5% dysthymia	Significantly higher prevalence in patients with late stage disease
Nuhu et al. [66]	210	Various cancer sites; Nigerian cohort	SCID interview, MADRS	30% major depression	
Mhaidat et al. [67]	208	Various cancer sites; Jordanian cohort	HADS	51.9% depressed	High prevalence of depression possibly related to negative perception of prognosis
Christensen et al. [68]	3321	Breast cancer; Danish cohort	BDI	13.7% major depression	
Den Oudsten et al. [69]	223	Breast cancer	CES-D	40.9% before diagnosis; 27.8% 1 yr later	

BDI, Beck Depression Inventory; BHS, Beck Hopelessness Scale; BSI, Brief Symptom Inventory; CES-D, Center for Epidemiology Self-report Depression Scale; DIS, Diagnostic Interview Schedule; EORTC-QLQ, European Organization for Research and Treatment of Cancer-Quality of Life Questionnaire; FLIC, Functional Living Index of Cancer; GAIS, Global Adjustment to Illness Scale; GHQ, General Health Questionnaire; HRSD, Hamilton Rating Scale for Depression; HADS, Hospital Anxiety and Depression Scale; HIS-GWB, Rand Health Insurance Study-General Well-Being Schedule; IBQ, Illness Behaviour Questionnaire; MADRS, Montgomery-Asberg Depression Rating Scale; MILP, Monash Interview for Liaison Psychiatry; MMPI, Minnesota Multiphasic Personality Inventory; MPAC, Memorial Pain Assessment Card; PHQ, Patient Health Questionnaire; POMS, Profile of Mood States; QOL, Quality of Life questionnaire; RDC, Research Diagnostic Criteria; RDS, Raskin Depression Screen; RSCL, Rotterdam Symptom Checklist; SCID, Structured Clinical Interview for DSM; SCL-25, SCL-90, SCL-90R, Hopkins Symptom Checklist 25, 90, and 90-Revised; SDS, Self-rated Depression Scale; SF-36, Medical Outcomes Study 36-Item Short Form Survey; STAI, State-Trait Anxiety Inventory.

A limitation of many studies is that the effects of cancer treatments and non-cancer related variables that affect mood are not accounted for. For example, although drugs can cause depression in some people, research groups usually have not presented data about cytotoxic drug or hormone use when describing their findings.

Several papers from Nemeroff's group [70–72] acknowledge the many reasons why it is difficult to compare studies (different definitions of depression, cancer type or stage, time since diagnosis, varying cancer treatments, personal history of depression and treatment for depression), but importantly, they underscore several general observations. The severity of medical illness, as manifested by significant pain, declining performance status, or the need for ongoing treatment, is associated with a high risk of comorbid depression. Whether high rates of depression associated with some cancers are due to the pathophysiologic effect of the tumour (i.e. cytokine or paraneoplastic syndromes associated with breast, pancreas, testis or lung cancers), treatment effects or other unidentified factors remain to be discerned. Nonetheless, we confidently conclude that cancer, exclusive of site, is associated with a rate of depression that is higher than in the general population.

Cancer types highly associated with depression include brain (41–93%) [57, 63], pancreas (up to 50%) [11], head and neck (up to 42%) [52], breast (4.5–37%) [45, 55], gynaecological (23%) [74] and lung (11%) [40]. A large cross-sectional study of 8265 adult outpatients revealed higher levels of mixed anxiety/depression symptoms in patients with stomach (20%), pancreatic (17%), head and neck (15%) and lung (14%) cancers [73]. A lower prevalence of depression is reported in patients with other cancers, such as colon (13%) [11] and lymphoma (8%) [19].

DeFlorio and Massie reviewed 49 studies of the prevalence of depression in individuals with cancer with a particular emphasis on gender differences [75]. Twenty-three studies found no gender differences in the prevalence of depression at a significance level of $p < 0.05$. However, 10 research groups found either gender differences in subsets of patients, non-significant trends, or differences in other parameters such as psychiatric morbidity, anxiety and denial.

In their study of 808 cancer patients, Kathol *et al.* [26] found women were more depressed than men using Research Diagnostic Criteria;

however, this finding did not persist when DSM-III criteria were applied. Sneed *et al.* [31] found no gender differences in depression, anxiety, hostility, somatization, general psychological distress, or psychological well-being. Fife *et al.* [76] also found no significant differences in depression in male and female cancer patients; however, they found that women made a more positive adjustment to cancer.

DEPRESSION BY CANCER TYPE

Depression in Women with Breast Cancer

Breast cancer is the cancer most studied in terms of psychosocial effects. The reported prevalence of depression ranges from 4.5% to 37%. One of the larger studies [68], examining 3321 early stage Danish breast cancer patients, recently found a 13.7% prevalence of major depression 12–16 weeks after surgery (17.9% in 18–35 year olds and 11.2% in 60–69 year olds). Independent risk factors for the development of depression included younger age, social status, ethnicity, comorbidity, psychiatric history, physical functioning, smoking, alcohol use and body mass index (BMI). Kissane *et al.* [39], in 303 early stage and 200 metastatic breast cancer patients, found prevalence rates of major depression of 9.6 and 6.5% respectively. Fatigue, a past history of depression, and cognitive attitudes of helplessness, hopelessness or resignation were significantly associated with depression in both groups.

Some research groups have assessed the duration of psychological distress in breast cancer patients. In a prospective study of 160 women awaiting breast surgery, Morris *et al.* [12] found a 22% prevalence of depression in women who had a mastectomy for breast cancer. This prevalence persisted at two years, compared to an 8% prevalence of depression in those with benign disease. One five-year observational cohort study of 222 early stage breast cancer patients [77] revealed prevalence rates for depression and anxiety of 33% at diagnosis, 15% after one year and 45% after a recurrence was diagnosed.

Few researchers have correlated patients' history of depression with current depression and/or functioning. In a study of 303 relatively young (mean age 46) women with early (Stage I or II) breast cancer at

3 months after breast surgery, using a structured diagnostic interview, Kissane *et al.* [39] found that a past history of depression was associated with current depression. They also noted that women with few psychological symptoms and good emotional adjustment to cancer may have refused participation in the study, because these women were also being recruited into an intervention study. Pasacreta [78] reported findings on a homogenous sample of 79 women evaluated with the Diagnostic Interview Schedule and the Center for Epidemiological Studies Depression Scale, three–seven months after their diagnosis of breast cancer. Women with elevated depressive symptoms had more physical symptom distress and more impaired functioning than subjects without depression.

Depression in Women with Gynaecological Cancer

In a systematic review which included 18 studies of psychological distress in ovarian cancer patients, Arden-Close *et al.* [79] found strong evidence for a relationship of younger age, more advanced disease at diagnosis, more physical symptoms and shorter time since diagnosis with increased levels of anxiety and/or depression. In the 12 studies rated as methodologically good, 21–25% of patients scored above the clinical cut-off for depression. In examining depression in ovarian cancer patients, Goncalves *et al.* [80] noted that persistent clinical depression tended to be not prevalent (6%), and that the highest prevalence was at the beginning of treatment. Neuroticism and the use of antidepressants were independent predictors of depression. For women with gynaecologic cancer, Evans *et al.* [74] found a 23% prevalence of depression and a 24% prevalence of adjustment disorder with depressed mood.

Depression in Patients with Head and Neck Cancer

Head and neck malignancies carry high risks of morbidity and mortality, with disease and treatment factors contributing substantially to disfigurement and loss of vital functions, such as eating, breathing and communicating. A systematic review of 52 studies found that depression is present throughout the trajectory of illness in patients with oropharyngeal cancers. Depression rates were highest at the time of diagnosis (13–40%), during treatment (25–52%), and at six-month follow-up (11–45%); the levels decreased three years after diagnosis (9–27%) [81]. Other correlates of depression in this review included: patient characteristics (male, unmarried, less education, history of past and current smoking, young age, lower physical functioning and low social supports); patient physical symptoms (pain, fatigue, insomnia and anorexia); and treatment characteristics (combined and aggressive treatments).

de Leeuw *et al.* assessed the predictive values of numerous pre-treatment variables [52]. Tumour stage, gender, depressive symptoms, openness to discuss cancer in the family, available support, received emotional support, tumour related symptoms, and size of an informal social network were calculated six months to three years after treatment. They concluded that these variables could be used to accurately predict which head and neck cancer patients were more likely to become depressed up to three years after treatment.

Hammerlid *et al.* [41], studying 357 head and neck cancer patients, found that those who reported a higher level of mental distress had lower performance status and more advanced disease.

Depression in Patients with Lung Cancer

Lung cancer has often been associated with higher levels of distress and depression than other tumour sites. In a study of depression and anxiety in 129 lung cancer patients, before and after diagnosis, Montazeri *et al.* [40] found that 10% of patients had severe anxiety symptoms and 12% had symptoms of depression at first presentation to their pulmonary physician. Depression, but not anxiety, increased by 10% at follow-up. Hopwood and Stephens [45] studied 987 lung cancer patients and found that depression was common and persistent, and that it was more prevalent for those patients with more severe symptoms and functional limitations. Depression was also more prevalent in patients with small cell lung cancer than non-small cell lung cancer.

In a study of 129 newly diagnosed patients with non-small cell lung cancer, using a clinical interview that generated a DSM diagnosis, Akechi *et al.* [50] reported a high prevalence of mental disorders. The most common psychiatric disorder at baseline was nicotine dependence (67%), followed by adjustment disorders (14%), alcohol dependence (13%), and major depression (5%).

Depression in Patients Undergoing Stem-Cell Transplantation

Loberiza *et al.* [82] prospectively studied 193 adults who received autologous or allogenic hematopoietic stem-cell transplantation using the Short Form-36 and the Spitzer Quality of Life Index Scale. The authors controlled for patient, disease and transplantation prognostic factors, but unfortunately, no standardized measure of depression was utilized. Thirty-five per cent of the patients satisfied the authors' criteria for depressive syndrome, which was associated with high mortality in the 6–12 month period after transplantation.

Depression in Brain Tumours

In addition to the difficulty adjusting to an illness that contributes to considerable morbidity and mortality, psychiatric problems in brain tumour patients can also be directly caused by the disease process as well as by treatment, including chemotherapy, radiation and corti-costeroids. Arnold *et al.* [63] found that 41% of 363 brain tumour patients had depressive symptoms, as assessed by a modified version of the Brief Patient Health Questionnaire. Female gender, lower education, lower tumour grade and previous psychiatric disorder were predictors of depression. Although not significant, being unmarried and having a past/current medical illness trended toward being predictors of depression. Although based on symptoms, Litofsky *et al.* [57] found that 93% of 598 high-grade glioma patients reported depressive symptoms in the early post-operative period, compared to 15% recognized by their physicians, highlighting the potential for underdiagnosis of depression in this population. Of 60 brain tumour patients, Pelletier *et al.* [83] found that 38% scored in the clinically depressed range on the Beck Depressive Inventory-II. Although depression, fatigue, emotional distress and existential problems were interrelated, depression was the most important independent predictor of quality of life, emphasizing the importance of its recognition and treatment.

Depression in Patients with Lymphoma, Pancreatic, Gastric and Colon Cancer

Studies of the prevalence of depression in adults with lymphoma, pancreatic, gastric and colon cancers are fewer in number [84]. Wide ranges in the reported prevalence of depression are noted but, in general, patients with lymphoma, gastric and colon cancer have a lower prevalence of depression than those with pancreatic cancer.

DEPRESSION IN ADVANCED CANCER AND PALLIATIVE CARE

Depression is common in patients with advanced cancer [85], yet all too often remains underdiagnosed and undertreated [86]. The barriers facing healthcare professionals in this area are considerable. One of them is the common misconception that it is normal for patients with advanced cancer to be sad. Yet, despite such barriers, we must not lose sight of the fact that depression is an independent predictor of poor survival in advanced cancer [87]. Furthermore, it reduces quality of life and prolongs hospitalization [88]. Most importantly, depression in advanced cancer is treatable, and validated assessment tools have been developed to facilitate diagnosis.

Due to variation in diagnostic criteria, prevalence estimates vary widely from 5 to 26% for major depression and from 7 to 26% for minor depression in those with advanced cancer [89–91]. The highest prevalence rates of depression have been observed in patients with cancers of the pancreas, head and neck, and breast [92]. Brintzenhofe-Szoc *et al.* [73] conducted a large cross-sectional study in an outpatient setting to determine the cancer specific prevalence of both pure depression and mixed anxiety/depression. The highest prevalence of pure depression was in patients with pancreatic cancer, while the highest prevalence of mixed anxiety/depression was in those with cancer of the stomach.

A past history of depression is the greatest risk factor for developing major depression in advanced cancer [90]. Pain, poor functional status, limited social network and younger age are also important risk factors [91]. Psychological concomitants promoting depression include the emotional impact of the advanced diagnosis, medication side effects, progression of cancer with its associated disability, and cerebral dysfunction [92].

Depression in advanced cancer not only reduces quality of life, but also shortens survival time, reduces compliance with treatment and prolongs hospitalization [87, 93, 94]. It also places a considerable psychological burden on carers and family members [95]. It can lead to a desire to hasten death in terminally ill cancer patients [96, 97]. Recent studies have suggested that depression is not only associated with interest in physician-assisted suicide, but also instability of this interest. When confronted with a request for assisted suicide, the possibility of depression should always be considered [98].

There are no universally accepted criteria for diagnosing depression in the terminally ill patient. Given the neurovegetative features associated with advanced cancer, difficulties arise when deciding which of the somatic symptoms identified in the DSM-IV criteria are attributable to depression and which are due to cancer [93]. Endicott suggested that the somatic symptoms should be replaced by other criteria in the cancer setting [94]. Others encourage an inclusive approach to somatic symptoms if they are severe and proportionate to the illness [99].

Patients often find it difficult to disclose emotional concerns with medical professionals, who themselves may find it difficult to raise such issues [97, 100]. As a result, depression frequently goes undetected in advanced cancer. Given these difficulties, there has been an increasing interest in the development of assessment tools [101]. Such screening instruments are not diagnostic and only serve to identify those patients with symptoms suggestive of depression. When patients are identified by screening, further assessment may be required before treatment is commenced.

Although there remains no ideal screening questionnaire for identifying depression in advanced cancer, the Hospital Anxiety and Depression scale (HADS) devised by Zigmond and Snaith [102] remains one of the most widely used tools. The HADS is a concise, self-reported questionnaire with 14 items, and was originally intended as a screening tool for medical patients. The HADS excludes physical and emotional indicators of depression and instead focuses on those relating to anhedonia – the inability to experience pleasure from normally pleasurable experiences. Although the HADS appears to perform well in those receiving active anti-cancer treatment, it performs less well in those with progressive disease [103]. This in turn results in a limited sensitivity and specificity when the HADS is used alone as a screening tool [104].

The Edinburgh Depression Scale (EDS), an assessment tool originally designed to screen for postnatal depression in the community, has also shown much promise [105]. This tool also excludes somatic symptoms of depression and replaces those with questions on worthlessness, subjective sadness, and suicidal ideation. The inclusion of questions relating to self harm may be particularly discriminating and represents an independent indicator of depression [106]. One study of palliative care patients using the EDS found that a cut-off threshold of 13 had a sensitivity of 0.79, a specificity of 0.81 and a positive predictive value of 0.53 using ICD-10 criteria for depression [107]. This compares with a sensitivity of 0.77 and a specificity of 0.85 for the HAD scale [108]. More recently, a Brief Edinburgh Depression Scale (BEDS) has been validated, which is more discriminating for depression in patients with advanced cancer than the original 10-item scale. The BEDS has a sensitivity of 0.72, a specificity of 0.83 and a positive predictive value of 0.65 [109]. This tool is now widely used in the palliative care setting when screening for depression [87].

There is strong evidence to suggest that depression is not only underdiagnosed but also undertreated in advanced cancer [110]. There remains a weak correlation between detection of a depressive disorder and actual treatment [111]. The single most important barrier to treatment is the common misconception that it is normal for patients with advanced cancer to be sad. Other barriers to effective treatment of depression in advanced cancer include pre-conceived ideas that psychological treatment is better than pharmacological measures, and attitudes of therapeutic nihilism, that is, nothing works at this stage [112]. In those situations where antidepressant medication is commenced, it is frequently done so at inadequate doses or too late for a therapeutic effect to take place [113]. One survey conducted in UK palliative care units found that 76% of antidepressants were started in the last two weeks of life [113].

DEMORALIZATION

Despite the increasing focus on mood disorders in cancer care, the role of meaning in understanding the illness experience has been somewhat neglected. Here the concept of demoralization comes to the fore. Frank [114] described demoralization as a persistent inability to cope, together with feelings of helplessness, hopelessness, meaninglessness, subjective incompetence and diminished self-esteem. Obviously, depression and demoralization are closely related, both in their phenomenology and our understanding of how they develop. Although demoralization may be a precursor or even co-exist with depression, the two are essentially different constructs. The central feature of depression is pervasive anhedonia and a loss of consummatory pleasure in the present moment. This contrasts with demoralization, where the individual retains the capacity to enjoy the present moment, but the future is perceived to be without value – there is a loss of anticipatory pleasure [115]. The demoralized feel inhibited in action by not knowing what to do, feeling helpless and incompetent; the depressed have lost motivation and drive even when an appropriate direction of action is known.

Frankl [116] noted that, for life to have meaning, it must offer the experience of self-transcendence. He recognized that meaning can also be found in suffering by transcending the moment to understand the fullest impact of the experience. Engel [117] presented lucid descriptions of demoralization in his 'giving up-given up syndrome'. While studying psychological states that predispose people to become sick, he and his colleagues observed this syndrome, which was thought to precede physical illness. This was commonly precipitated by a loss and was characterized by a physiological slowing of bodily functions such as reduced heart rate and the affects of helplessness and hopelessness. But does physical illness lead to demoralization or vice versa? The available evidence appears to suggest that both may occur [118]. Frank emphasized the central importance of mobilizing hope to induce healing and described a restoration of morale as the critical aspect underpinning success [114].

Although several possible diagnostic criteria have been proposed for demoralization, it has not yet been defined in the DSM. de Figueiredo [119] highlighted that, in this multi-axial system, demoralization includes symptoms of anxiety and depressive disorders (axis I), is affected by personality traits (axis II), is clearly to be associated with physical health problems (axis III) and is related to the level of functioning (axis V). Many demoralized individuals are inadequately labelled as suffering from 'adjustment disorders' for lack of a better term and to satisfy third-party payers who demand a diagnostic label. This type of confusion occurs because our current diagnostic systems fail to recognize four perspectives of every person: his/her disease, behaviour, illness and life story. Demoralization is intimately related to a person's life story. One suggestion was made that demoralization could replace stressful life events in axis IV [119]. But such events are circumstances that are external to the individual, and simply listing them under axis IV, or reducing demoralization to a V-code, tells us nothing about the internal struggle of the person exposed to the stress [120].

Morale can vary across a spectrum of mental attitudes, ranging from disheartenment (a mild loss of confidence) to despondency (starting to give up) and despair (losing hope), before eventually reaching the state of demoralization (having given up) [121]. Whilst the initial stages of this spectrum represent a comprehensible response to adversity, the later stages are pathological through their maladaptiveness, the extent of personal distress and the potential to generate greater harm through further deterioration.

Kissane *et al.* [121] emphasized the clinical importance of demoralization as a concept. Contrary to the original definition of Frank, Clarke and Kissane's review [122] concluded that demoralization can be distinct from depression – depressed patients experience anhedonia, whereas demoralized patients experience subjective incompetence. Kissane *et al.* [121] proposed criteria for the demoralization syndrome (see Table 1.2).

This concept was aided by the development of a tool to measure demoralization, the Demoralization Scale [123]. In a cohort of

Table 1.2 Proposed diagnostic criteria for the demoralization syndrome (adapted from Kissane *et al.* [122]).

A. Affective symptoms of existential distress including loss of meaning and purpose in life or hopelessness
B. Cognitive attitudes of pessimism, helplessness, sense of being trapped, personal failure, or lacking a worthwhile future
C. Conative absence of motivation to cope differently
D. Associated features of social alienation or isolation and lack of support
E. Allowing for fluctuation in emotional intensity, these phenomena persist across more than two weeks
F. A major depressive or other psychiatric disorder is not present as the primary condition

patients with advanced cancer, this 24-item, self-report questionnaire demonstrated good reliability and strong concurrent validity with measures of existential distress, hopelessness and depression. Of particular interest was the observation that the two items closest in content to suicidal ideation, 'life is no longer worth living' and 'I would rather not be alive', load strongly on the loss of meaning subscale. The dimensions of the phenomenology of demoralization are captured in the tool's subscales: dysphoria, disheartenment, loss of meaning, helplessness and sense of failure. Other cohorts of palliative care patients have permitted the differentiation of depression with anhedonia from depression with demoralization [124].

Clarke *et al.* [125] compared 125 patients with metastatic cancer and 126 patients with motor neurone disease (MND) on a range of physical and psychosocial measures as they approached the end of life. The MND patients were younger, had greater social contacts, but were more physically impaired, while the cancer patients had more pain and were on more medication (opioids, steroids, and other analgesics). Although the Beck Depression Inventory scores were similar in the two groups, MND patients had significantly higher scores for demoralization, hopelessness, and suicidal ideation. Cancer patients, on the other hand, scored significantly higher on anhedonia. This difference in the quality of depression was argued to represent a difference in illness experience of the two groups, which has relevance for the ways we treat depression in the medically ill.

The concept of demoralization clearly has profound implications for clinical practice [126, 127]. Recent evidence suggests that, when allowance is made for demoralization to be comorbidly present with depression, prevalence rates between 20 and 30% for demoralization are seen across studies, with higher rates in advanced cancer than in early cancer states [128]. In the UK, a multi-centre, longitudinal study into the prevalence of depression and demoralization in patients with advanced cancer has recently been undertaken by Lloyd-Williams *et al.* A sample of 629 patients, aged from 21 to 94 years, was recruited from hospice and palliative care day units in the northern part of England and parts of North Wales. Thirty-two per cent of patients had a diagnosis of breast cancer, 17% of gastrointestinal cancers and 17% cancers of the lung; 67% were female. On Eastern Cooperative Oncology Group (ECOG) performance scores, 69% had scores of 1 or 2, indicating that they were ambulatory patients. Thirty-four per cent of the cohort stated they had experienced depression previously and 32% of participants scored 10 or more on the Patient Health Questionnaire, indicating a diagnosis of major depression. Patients also completed the Royal Free Spirituality Scale. Preliminary findings confirm that demoralization and depression are strongly positively correlated, while negatively correlated with spiritually. Spirituality appears to provide the meaning to counter demoralization.

CONCLUSIONS

Depression is common in adults with cancer, and frequently co-exists with anxiety and pain. It has been challenging to study because symptoms occur on a spectrum that ranges from sadness to major affective disorder, and mood change is often difficult to evaluate when a patient is confronted by repeated threats to life, is receiving complex cancer treatments, is fatigued, and/or is experiencing pain. Untreated depression, nevertheless, results in significant morbidity and mortality. Although the prevalence of depression varies across the 60 studies of at least 100 cancer patients cited in this chapter, ranging between 1.5 and 52%, there should be no doubt that cancer is associated with a high degree of depression.

Depression is especially common in patients with advanced cancer, in whom it is frequently missed and therefore not treated. The diagnosis of depression in this population represents a particular challenge given the vegetative features associated with advanced cancer. The impact of the illness on the morale of the patients allows insight to be gained into sources of meaning in their life, which informs the choice of treatment.

Future research must focus on establishing diagnostically reliable criteria, developing standard instruments for measuring depression, correlating past psychiatric history of depression and anxiety with current mood, characterising the causative role of antineoplastics in depression, and identifying biological markers for depression. There is much to do to enhance the quality of life of patients with cancer and prevent the onset of depression.

REFERENCES

1. Kessler, R.C., Berglund, P., Demler, O. *et al.* (2003) The epidemiology of major depressive disorder. Results from the National Comorbidity Survey Replication (NCS-R). *JAMA*, **289**, 3095–3105.
2. Grady-Weliky, T.A. (2002) Comorbidity and its implication on treatment: change over the life span. Presented at the American Psychiatric Association Annual Meeting. Philadelphia, May 2002.
3. Seedat, S., Scott, K.M., Angermeyer, M.C. *et al.* (2009) Cross-national associations between gender and mental disorders in the World Health Organization World Mental Health Surveys. *Arch. Gen. Psychiatry*, **66**, 785–795.
4. Katon, W., Lin, E.H. and Kroenke, K. (2007) The association of depression and anxiety with medical symptom burden in patients with chronic medical illness. *Gen. Hosp. Psychiatry*, **29**, 147–155.
5. Massie, M.J. and Popkin, M.K. (1998) Depressive disorders, in *PsychoOncology* (ed. J.C. Holland), Oxford University Press, New York, pp. 514–540.
6. Wallen, J., Pincus, H.A., Goldman, H.H. and Marcus, S.E. (1987) Psychiatric consultations in short-term general hospitals. *Arch. Gen. Psychiatry*, **44**, 163–168.
7. Snyder, S., Strain, J.J. and Wolf, D. (1987) Differentiating major depression from adjustment disorder with depressed mood in the medical setting. *Gen. Hosp. Psychiatry*, **12**, 159–165.

8. Wells, K.B., Golding, J.M. and Burham, M.A. (1988) Psychiatric disorder in a sample of the general population with and without chronic medical conditions. *Am. J. Psychiatry*, **145**, 976–981.

9. Popkin, M.K. and Tucker, G.J. (1994) Mental disorders due to a general medical condition and substance-induced disorders; mood anxiety, psychotic, and personality disorders, in *DSM-IV Sourcebook*, vol. **1** (eds T.A. Widiger, A.J. Frances, H.A., Pincus *et al.*), American Psychiatric Association, Washington, pp. 243–276.

10. Derogatis, L.R., Morrow, G.R. and Fetting, J. (1983) The prevalence of psychiatric disorders among cancer patients. *JAMA*, **249**, 751–757.

11. Fras, I., Litin, E. and Pearson, J.S. (1967) Comparison of psychiatric symptoms in carcinoma of the pancreas with those in some other intra-abdominal neoplasm. *Am. J. Psychiatry*, **123**, 1553–1562.

12. Morris, T., Greer, H.S. and White, P. (1977) Psychological and social adjustment to mastectomy. *Cancer*, **40**, 2381.

13. Maguire, G.P., Lee, E., Bevington, D. *et al.* (1978) Psychiatric problems in the first year after mastectomy. *BMJ*, **1**, 963–965.

14. Silberfarb, P.M., Maurer, L.H. and Crouthamel, C.S. (1980) Psychological aspects of neoplastic disease: I. Functional status of breast cancer patients during different treatment regimens. *Am. J. Psychiatry*, **137**, 450–455.

15. Farber, J.M., Weinerman, B.H. and Kuypers, J.A. (1984) Psychosocial distress in oncology outpatients. *J. Psychosoc. Oncol.*, **2**, 109–118.

16. Hughes, J.E. (1985) Depressive illness and lung cancer. I. Depression before diagnosis. *Eur. J. Surg. Oncol.*, **11**, 15–20.

17. Lansky, S.B., List, M.A., Herrmann, C.A. *et al.* (1985) Absence of major depressive disorder in female cancer patients. *J. Clin. Oncol.*, **3**, 1553–1560.

18. Holland, J.C., Korzan, A.H., Tross, S. *et al.* (1986) Comparative psychological disturbance in patients with pancreatic and gastric cancer. *Am. J. Psychiatry*, **143**, 982–986.

19. Devlen, J., Maguire, P., Phillips, P. and Crowther, D. (1987) Psychological problems associated with diagnosis and treatment of lymphoma. II: Prospective study. *BMJ*, **295**, 955–957.

20. Larsy, J.C.M., Margolese, R.G., Poisson, R. *et al.* (1987) Depression and body image following mastectomy and lumpectomy. *J. Chronic Dis.*, **40**, 529–534.

21. Stefanek, M.E., Derogatis, L.P. and Shaw, A. (1987) Psychological distress among oncology outpatients. *Psychosomatics*, **28**, 530539.

22. Pettingale, K.W., Burgess, C. and Greer, S. (1987) Psychological response to cancer diagnosis - I. Correlations with prognostic variables. *J. Psychosom. Res.*, **32**, 255–261.

23. Grassi, L., Rosti, G., Albieri, G. and Marangolo, M. (1989) Depression and abnormal illness behavior in cancer patients. *Gen. Hosp. Psychiatry*, **11**, 404–411.
24. Hardman, A., Maguire, P. and Crowther, D. (1989) The recognition of psychiatric morbidity on a medical oncology ward. *J. Psychosom. Res.*, **33**, 235–239.
25. Fallowfield, L.J., Hall, A., Maguire, G.P. and Baum, M. (1990) Psychological outcomes of different treatment policies in women with early breast cancer outside of a clinical trial. *BMJ*, **301**, 575–580.
26. Kathol, R., Mutgi, A., Williams, J. *et al.* (1990) Diagnosis of major depression according to four sets of criteria. *Am. J. Psychiatry*, **147**, 1021–1024.
27. Colon, E.A., Callies, A.L., Popkin, M.K. and McGlave, P.B. (1991) Depressed mood and other variables related to bone marrow transplantation survival in acute leukemia. *Psychosomatics*, **32**, 420–425.
28. Hopwood, P., Howell, A. and Maquire, P. (1991) Psychiatric morbidity in patients with advanced cancer of the breast: prevalence measured to two self-rating questionnaires. *Br. J. Cancer*, **64**, 349–352.
29. Goldberg, J.A., Scott, R.N. and Davidson, P.M. (1992) Psychological morbidity in the first year after breast surgery. *Eur. J. Surg. Oncol.*, **18**, 327–331.
30. Maraste, R., Brandt, L., Olson, H. and Ryde-Brandt, B. (1992) Anxiety and depression in breast cancer patients at start of adjuvant radiotherapy. *Acta Oncol.*, **31**, 641–643.
31. Sneed, N.V., Edlund, B. and Dias, J.K. (1992) Adjustment of gynecological and breast cancer patients to the cancer diagnosis: comparisons with males and females having other cancer sites. *Health Care Women Intl.*, **13**, 11–22.
32. Carroll, B.T., Kathol, R.G., Noyes, R. *et al.* (1993) Screening for depression and anxiety in cancer patients using the Hospital Anxiety and Depression Scale. *Gen. Hosp. Psychiatry*, **15**, 69–74.
33. Cathcart, C.K., Jones, S.E., Pumroy, C.S. *et al.* (1993) Clinical recognition and management of depression in node negative breast cancer patients treated with tamoxifen. *Breast Cancer Res. Treat.*, **27**, 277–281.
34. Pinder, K.L., Ramirez, A.J. and Black, M.E. (1993) Psychiatric disorder in patients with advanced breast cancer: prevalence and associated factors. *Eur. J. Cancer*, **29**, 524–527.
35. Sneeuw, K.C.A., Aaronson, N.K., van Wouwe, M.C.C. *et al.* (1992) Prevalence and screening of psychiatric disorder in patients with early stage breast cancer. Presented at the International Congress of Psychosocial Oncology, Beaune, October 1992.

36. Kelsen, D.P., Portenoy, R.K., Thaler, H.T. *et al.* (1995) Pain and depression in patients with newly diagnosed pancreas cancer. *J. Clin. Oncol.*, **13**, 748–755.

37. Aass, N., Fossa, S.D., Dahl, A.A. and Moe, T.J. (1997) Prevalence of anxiety and depression in cancer patients seen at the Norwegian Radium Hospital. *Eur. J. Cancer*, **33**, 1597–1604.

38. Berard, R.M.F., Boermeester, F. and Viljoen, G. (1998) Depressive disorders in an out-patient oncology setting: prevalence, assessment and management. *Psychooncology*, **7**, 112–120.

39. Kissane, D.W., Clarke, D.M., Ikin, J. *et al.* (1998) Psychological morbidity and quality of life in Australian women with early-stage breast cancer: a cross-sectional survey. *Med. J. Australia*, **169**, 192–196.

40. Montazeri, A., Milroy, R., Hole, D. *et al.* (1998) Anxiety and depression in patients with lung cancer before and after diagnosis: findings from a population in Glasgow, Scotland. *J. Epidemiol. Community Health*, **52**, 203–204.

41. Hammerlid, E., Ahiner-Elmqvist, M., Bjordal, K. *et al.* (1999) A prospective multicentre study in Sweden and Norway of mental distress and psychiatric morbidity in head and neck cancer patients. *Br. J. Cancer*, **80**, 766–774.

42. Bodurka-Bevers, D., Basen-Engquist, K., Carmack, C.L. *et al.* (2000) Depression, anxiety, and quality of life in patients with epithelial ovarian cancer. *Gynecol. Oncol.*, **78**, 302–308.

43. Chen, M., Chang, H. and Yeh, C. (2000) Anxiety and depression in Taiwanese cancer patients with and without pain. *J. Adv. Cancer*, **32**, 944–951.

44. De Leeuw, J.R.J., de Graeff, A., Ros, W.J.G. *et al.* (2000) Negative and positive influences of social support on depression in patients with head and neck cancer: a prospective study. *Psychooncology*, **9**, 20–28.

45. Hopwood, P. and Stephens, R.J. (2000) Depression in patients with lung cancer: prevalence and risk factors derived from quality-of-life data. *J. Clin. Oncol.*, **18**, 893–903.

46. Kugaya, A., Akechi, T., Okuyama, T. *et al.* (2000) Prevalence, predictive factors, and screening for psychologic distress in patients with newly diagnosed head and neck cancer. *Cancer*, **88**, 2817–2823.

47. Pascoe, S., Edelman, S. and Kidman, A. (2000) Prevalence of psychological distress and use of support services by cancer patients at Sydney hospitals. *Aust. N. Z. J. Psychiatry*, **34**, 785–791.

48. Skarstein, J., Aass, N., Fossa, S.D. *et al.* (2000) Anxiety and depression in cancer patients: relation between the Hospital Anxiety and Depression Scale and the European Organization for Research and Treatment

of Cancer Core Quality of Life Questionnaire. *J. Psychosom. Res.*, **49**, 27–34.

49. Akechi, T., Okuyama, T., Imoyo, S. *et al.* (2001) Biomedical and psychosocial determinants of psychiatric morbidity among postoperative ambulatory breast cancer patients. *Breast Cancer Res. Treat.*, **65**, 195–202.

50. Akechi, T., Okamura, H., Nishiwaki, Y. and Uchitomi, Y. (2001) Psychiatric disorders and associated and predictive factors in patients with unresectable non small cell lung carcinoma. *Cancer*, **92**, 2609–2622.

51. Ciaramella, A. and Poli, P. (2001) Assessment of depression among cancer patients: the role of pain, cancer type and treatment. *Psychooncology*, **10**, 156–165.

52. De Leeuw, J.R.J., de Graeff, A., Ros, W.J.G. *et al.* (2001) Prediction of depression 6 months to 3 years after treatment of head and neck cancer. *Head Neck*, **23**, 892–898.

53. Sharpe, M., Strong, V., Allen, K. *et al.* (2004) Major depression in outpatients attending a regional cancer centre: screening and unmet treatment needs. *Br. J. Cancer*, **90**, 314–320.

54. Atesci, F.C., Baltalarli, B., Oguzhanoglu, N.K. *et al.* (2004) Psychiatric morbidity among cancer patients and awareness of illness. *Support. Care Cancer*, **12**, 161–167.

55. Kissane, D.W., Grabsch, B., Love, A. *et al.* (2004) Psychiatric disorder in women with early stage and advanced breast cancer: a comparative analysis. *Aust. N. Z. J. Psychiatry*, **38**, 320–326.

56. Nan, K.J., Wei, Y.C., Zhou, F. *et al.* (2004) Effects of depression on parameters of cell-mediated immunity in patients with digestive tract cancers. *World J. Gastroenterol.*, **10**, 268–272.

57. Litofsky, N.S., Farace, E., Anderson, F. *et al.* (2004) Depression in patients with high-grade glioma: results of the glioma outcomes project. *Neurosurgery*, **54**, 358–367.

58. Thomas, B.C., Devi, N., Sarita, G.P. *et al.* (2005) Reliability and validity of the Malayalam Hospital Anxiety and Depression Scale (HADS) in cancer patients. *Indian J. Med. Res.*, **122**, 395–399.

59. Montazeri, A., Sajadian, A., Ebrahimi, M. and Akbari, M.E. (2005) Depression and the use of complementary medicine among breast cancer patients. *Support. Care Cancer*, **13**, 339–342.

60. Wedding, U., Koch, A., Rohrig, B. *et al.* (2007) Requestioning depression in patients with cancer: contribution of somatic and affective symptoms to Beck's Depression Inventory. *Ann. Oncol.*, **18**, 1875–1881.

61. Steel, J.L., Geller, D.A., Gamblin, T.C. *et al.* (2007) Depression, immunity, and survival in patients with hepatobiliary carcinoma. *J. Clin. Oncol.*, **25**, 2397–2405.

62. Lueboonthavatchai, P. (2007) Prevalence and psychosocial factors of anxiety and depression in breast cancer patients. *J. Med. Assoc. Thai.*, **90**, 2164–2174.

63. Arnold, S.D., Forman, L.M., Brigidi, B.D. *et al.* (2008) Evaluation and characterization of generalized anxiety and depression in patients with primary brain tumors. *Neuro-oncology*, **10**, 171–181.

64. Wedding, U., Koch, A., Rohrig, B. *et al.* (2008) Depression and functional impairment independently contribute to decreased quality of life in cancer patients prior to chemotherapy. *Acta Oncol.*, **47**, 56–62.

65. Singer, S., Danker, H., Dietz, A. *et al.* (2008) Screening for mental disorders in laryngeal cancer patients: a comparison of 6 methods. *Psychooncology*, **17**, 280–286.

66. Nuhu, F.T., Odejide, O.A., Adebayo, K.O. and Adejumo, O. (2008) Prevalence and predictors of depression in cancer patients in the University College Hospital Ibadon, Nigeria. *Hong Kong J. Psychiatry*, **18**, 107–114.

67. Mhaidat, N.M., Alzoubi, K.H., Al-Sweedan, S. and Alhusein, B.A. (2009) Prevalence of depression among cancer patients in Jordan: a national survey. *Support. Care Cancer*, **11**, 1403–1407.

68. Christensen, S., Zachariae, R., Jensen, A.B. *et al.* (2009) Prevalence and risk of depressive symptoms 3–4 months post-surgery in a nationwide cohort study of Danish women treated for early stage breast-cancer. *Breast Cancer Res. Treat.*, **113**, 339–355.

69. Den Oudsten, B.L., Van Heck, G.L., Van der Steeg, A.F.W. *et al.* (2009) Predictors of depressive symptoms 12 months after surgical treatment of early-stage breast cancer. *Psychooncology*, **11**, 1230–1237.

70. Newport, D.J. and Nemeroff, C.B. (1998) Assessment and treatment of depression in the cancer patient. *J. Psychosom. Res.*, **45**, 215–237.

71. McDaniel, J.S., Musselman, D.L., Porter, M.R. *et al.* (1995) Depression in patients with cancer. *Arch. Gen. Psychiatry*, **52**, 89–99.

72. McDaniel, S.J. and Nemeroff, C.B. (1993) Depression in the cancer patient: diagnostic, biological, and treatment aspects, in *Current and Emerging Issues in Cancer Pain: Research and Practice* (eds. R.C. Chapmanand, K.M. Foley), Raven Press, New York, pp. 1–19.

73. Brintzenhofe-Szoc, K.M., Levin, T., Li, Y. *et al.* (2009) Mixed anxiety/depression symptoms in a large cancer cohort: prevalence by cancer type. *Psychosomatics*, **50**, 383–391.

PREVALENCE OF DEPRESSION IN PEOPLE WITH CANCER   33

74. Evans, D.L., McCartney, C.F., Nemeroff, C.B. *et al.* (1986) Depression in women treated for gynecological cancer: clinical and neuroendocrine assessment. *Am. J. Psychiatry*, **143**, 447–451.
75. DeFlorio, M.L. and Massie, M.J. (1995) Review of depression in cancer: gender differences. *Depression*, **3**, 66–80.
76. Fife, B.L., Kennedy, V.N. and Robinson, L. (1994) Gender and adjustment to cancer: clinical applications. *J. Psychosoc. Oncol.*, **12**, 1–21.
77. Burgess, C., Cornelius, V., Love, S. *et al.* (2005) Depression and anxiety in women with early breast cancer: five year observational cohort study. *BMJ*, **330**, 702–707.
78. Pasacreta, N. (1997) Depressive phenomena, physical symptom distress, and functional status among women with breast cancer. *Nurs. Res.*, **46**, 214–221.
79. Arden-Close, E., Gidron, Y. and Moss-Morris, R. (2008) Psychological distress and its correlates in ovarian cancer: a systematic review. *Psychooncology*, **17**, 1061–1072.
80. Goncalves, V., Jayson, G. and Tarrier, N. (2008) A longitudinal investigation of psychological morbidity in patients with ovarian cancer. *Br. J. Cancer*, **99**, 1794–1801.
81. Haisfield-Wolfe, M.E., McGuire, D.B., Soeken, K. *et al.* (2009) Prevalence and correlates of depression among patients with head and neck cancer: a systematic review of implications for research. *Oncol. Nurs. Forum*, **36**, E107–E125.
82. Loberiza, F.R. Jr, Rizzo, J.D., Bredeson, C.N. *et al.* (2002) Association of depressive syndrome and early deaths among patients after stem-cell transplantation for malignant diseases. *J. Clin. Oncol.*, **20**, 2118–2126.
83. Pelletier, G., Verhoef, M.J., Khatri, N. and Hagen, N. (2002) Quality of life in brain tumor patients: the relative contributions of depression, fatigue, emotional distress, and existential issues. *J. Neurooncol.*, **57**, 41–49.
84. Massie, M.J. (2004) Prevalence of depression in patients with cancer. *J. Natl. Cancer Inst. Monogr.*, **32**, 57–71.
85. Minagawa, H., Uchitomi, Y., Yamawaki, S. and Ishitani, K. (1996) Psychiatric morbidity in terminally ill cancer patients – A prospective study. *Cancer*, **78**, 1131–1137.
86. Breitbart, W. (1995) Identifying patients at risk for, and treatment of major psychiatric complications of cancer. *Support. Care Cancer*, **3**, 45–60.
87. Lloyd-Williams, M., Shiels, C., Taylor, F. and Dennis, M. (2009) Depression – An independent predictor of early death in patients with advanced cancer. *J. Affect. Disord.*, **113**, 127–132.

88. Pelletier, G. (2002) Quality of life in brain tumor patients: the relative contributions of depression, fatigue, emotional distress, and existential issues. *J. Neurooncol.*, **57**, 41–49.
89. McDaniel, J.S., Musselman, D.L., Porter, M.R. *et al.* (1995) Depression in patients with cancer – diagnosis, biology, and treatment. *Arch. Gen. Psychiatry*, **52**, 89–99.
90. Kadan-Lottick, N.S., Vanderwerker, L.C., Block, S.D. *et al.* (2005) Psychiatric disorders and mental health service use in patients with advanced cancer – A report from the coping with cancer study. *Cancer*, **104**, 2872–2881.
91. Potash, M. and Breitbart, W. (2002) Affective disorders in advanced cancer. *Hematol. Oncol. Clin. N. Am.*, **16**, 671–700.
92. Greer, S. and Silberfarb, P.M. (1982) Psychological concomitants of cancer - current state of research. *Psychol. Med.*, **12**, 563–573.
93. Lloyd-Williams, M., Dennis, M. and Taylor, F. (2004) A prospective study to determine the association between physical symptoms and depression in patients with advanced cancer. *Palliative Med.*, **18**, 558–563.
94. Endicott, J. (1984) Measurement of depression in patients with cancer. *Cancer*, **53**, 2243–2248.
95. Cassileth, B.R., Lusk, E.J., Strouse, T.B. *et al.* (1985) A psychological analysis of cancer patients and their next-of-kin. *Cancer*, **55**, 72–76.
96. Lloyd-Williams, M. (2000) Difficulties in diagnosing and treating depression in the terminally ill cancer patient. *Postgrad. Med. J.*, **76**, 555–558.
97. Maguire, P. (1985) Barriers to psychological care of the dying. *BMJ*, **291**, 1711–1713.
98. Emanuel, E.J., Fairclough, D.L. and Emanuel, L.L. (2000) Attitudes and desires related to euthanasia and physician-assisted suicide among terminally ill patients and their caregivers. *JAMA*, **284**, 2460–2468.
99. Cavanaugh, S.V. (1984) Diagnosing depression in the hospitalized patient with chronic medical illness. *J. Clin. Psychiatry*, **45**, 13–17.
100. Barraclough, J. (1997) ABC of palliative care – Depression, anxiety, and confusion. *BMJ*, **315**, 1365–1368.
101. Power, D., Kelly, S. and Gilsenan, J. (1993) Suitable screening tests for cognitive impairment and depression in the terminally ill: a prospective prevalence study. *Palliative Med.*, **7**, 213–218.
102. Zigmond, A.S. and Snaith, R.P. (1983) The Hospital Anxiety and Depression scale. *Acta Psychiatr. Scand.*, **67**, 361–370.
103. Ibbotson, T., Maguire, P., Selby, P. *et al.* (1994) Screening for anxiety and depression in cancer patients - the effects of disease and treatment. *Eur. J. Cancer*, **30**, 37–40.

104. Lloyd-Williams, M., Friedman, T. and Rudd, N. (2001) An analysis of the validity of the Hospital Anxiety and Depression Scale as a screening tool in patients with advanced metastatic cancer. *J. Pain Symptom Manag.*, **22**, 990–996.

105. Cox, J.L., Holden, J.M. and Sagovsky, R. (1987) Detection of postnatal depression – development of the 10-item Edinburgh Postnatal Depression Scale. *Br. J. Psychiatry*, **150**, 782–786.

106. Lloyd-Williams, M., Spiller, J. and Ward, J. (2003) Which depression screening tools should be used in palliative care? *Palliative Med.*, **17**, 40–43.

107. Lloyd-Williams, M., Friedman, T. and Rudd, N. (2000) Criterion validation of the Edinburgh postnatal depression scale as a screening tool for depression in patients with advanced metastatic cancer. *J. Pain Symptom Manag.*, **20**, 259–265.

108. Le Fevre, P., Devereux, J., Smith, S. *et al.* (1999) Screening for psychiatric illness in the palliative care inpatient setting: a comparison between the Hospital Anxiety and Depression Scale and the General Health Questionnaire-12. *Palliative Med.*, **13**, 399–407.

109. Lloyd-Williams, M., Shiels, C. and Dowrick, C. (2007) The development of the Brief Edinburgh Depression Scale (BEDS) to screen for depression in patients with advanced cancer. *J. Affect. Disord.*, **99**, 259–264.

110. Goldberg, R. (1985) A survey of psychotropic drugs used in terminal cancer patients. *Psychosomatics*, **26**, 745–751.

111. Ashbury, F.D., Madlensky, L. and Raich, P. (2003) Antidepressant prescribing in community cancer care. *Support. Care Cancer*, **11**, 278–285.

112. Dwight-Johnson, M., Ell, K. and Lee, P.J. (2005) Can collaborative care address the needs of low-income Latinas with comorbid depression and cancer? Results from a randomized pilot study. *Psychosomatics*, **46**, 224–232.

113. Lloyd-Williams, M., Friedman, T. and Rudd, N. (1999) A survey of antidepressant prescribing in the terminally ill. *Palliative Med.*, **13**, 243–248.

114. Frank, J.B. (1993) *Persuasion and Healing: A Comparative Study of Psychotherapy*, Johns Hopkins University Press, Baltimore.

115. de Figueiredo, J.M. (1993) Depression and demoralization – phenomenological differences and research perspectives. *Compr. Psychiatry*, **34**, 308–311.

116. Frankl, V.E. (1973) *The Doctor and the Soul: From Psychotherapy to Logotherapy*, Vintage Books, New York.

117. Engel, G.L. (1967) A psychological setting of somatic disease – giving up – given up complex. *Proc. Roy. Soc. Med.*, **60**, 553.
118. Spiegel, D. and Kato, P.M. (1996) Psychosocial influences on cancer incidence and progression. *Harvard Rev. Psychiatry*, **4**, 10–26.
119. de Figueiredo, J.M. (2007) Demoralization and psychotherapy: a tribute to Jerome D. Frank, MD, PhD (1909–2005). *Psychother. Psychosom.*, **76**, 129–133.
120. de Figueiredo, J.M. (1983) Some issues in research on the epidemiology of demoralization. *Compr. Psychiatry*, **24**, 154–157.
121. Kissane, D.W., Clarke, D.M. and Street, A.F. (2001) Demoralization syndrome – a relevant psychiatric diagnosis for palliative care. *J. Palliative Care*, **17**, 12–21.
122. Clarke, D.M. and Kissane, D.W. (2002) Demoralization: its phenomenology and importance. *Aust. N. Z. J. Psychiatry*, **36**, 733–742.
123. Kissane, D.W., Wein, S., Love, A. *et al.* (2004) The demoralization scale: a report of its development and preliminary validation. *J. Palliative Care*, **20**, 269–276.
124. Clarke, D.M., Kissane, D.W., Trauer, T. and Smith, G.C. (2005) Demoralization, anhedonia and grief in patients with severe physical illness. *World Psychiatry*, **4**, 96–105.
125. Clarke, D.M., McLeod, J.E., Smith, G.C. *et al.* (2005) A comparison of psychosocial and physical functioning in patients with motor neurone disease and metastatic cancer. *J. Palliative Care*, **21**, 173–179.
126. Clarke, D.M., Cook, K.E., Coleman, K.J. and Smith, G.C. (2006) A qualitative examination of the experience of 'depression' in hospitalized medically ill patients. *Psychopathology*, **39**, 303–312.
127. Lloyd-Williams, M., Reeve, J. and Kissane, D. (2008) Distress in palliative care patients: developing patient-centred approaches to clinical management. *Eur. J. Cancer*, **44**, 1133–1138.
128. Mangelli, L., Fava, G.A., Grandi, S. *et al.* (2005) Assessing demoralization and depression in the setting of medical disease. *J. Clin. Psychiatry*, **66**, 391–394.

CHAPTER 2

Psychological Adaptation, Demoralization and Depression in People with Cancer

David M. Clarke

School of Psychology and Psychiatry, Monash University, Melbourne, VIC, Australia

Depression is common in people with cancer, although not uniformly common across all cancers and all stages of treatment. But, what causes depression in cancer? E. Cassel'l [1], in his book *The Nature of Suffering and the Goals of Medicine*, makes the point that, although it is important to recognize and acknowledge depression when it is present, we must not forget that 'affect is merely the outward expression of the injury ... and is not the injury itself'. It is a bit like having a rash. The rash is only the symptom of an underlying injury or disease. Depression is a sign that something is threatening the vitality of the organism. In cancer, the process is both biological and psychological.

This chapter will focus on psychological adaptation in people with cancer and on the three quite distinguishable syndromes of anhedonic depression, demoralization and grief arising as a reaction to having cancer.

Depression and Cancer Edited by David W. Kissane, Mario Maj and Norman Sartorius
© 2011 John Wiley & Sons, Ltd

ANHEDONIC DEPRESSION, DEMORALIZATION AND GRIEF IN PEOPLE WITH CANCER

A number of researchers have studied the emotional reactions of people with cancer. Greer and Watson [2] observed and described five characteristic responses of people to the development of cancer. These included anxious preoccupation and helplessness-hopelessness, particularly associated with negative emotions, avoidance and denial, fatalism and fighting spirit. Helplessness-hopelessness was shown to be related to early death and relapse in patients with early stage breast cancer [3].

Jacobsen *et al.* [4] assessed the symptoms of 242 cancer patients. Factor analysis identified a distinct demoralization/despair factor characterized by feelings of loss of control, loss of hope, a sense of failure, feeling life was a burden, and a loss of meaning.

Clarke *et al.* [5, 6] completed a series of studies describing the depressive psychopathology of people with physical illness generally, and with cancer particularly. They showed that there were three quite distinguishable syndromes of anhedonic depression, demoralization and grief. Anhedonic depression was characterized by the lack of ability to experience pleasure and a consequent loss of interest in things. Demoralization was characterized by feelings of helplessness and hopelessness; though there may be some diminishment of pleasure, there is not a loss of ability to experience pleasure in all circumstances. Grief was characterized by a sense of 'loss', accompanied by pangs (or waves) of grief and pining for that which was lost.

Anhedonia has a strong place in the phenomenology of depression. Though not a requisite for a diagnosis of DSM major depressive disorder, it has, together with its associated non-reactivity of mood, a central place in melancholia. Indeed, it has often been considered the central feature of the most definable form of clinical depression, termed 'endogenomorphic depression' by D. Klein, which he describes as follows: 'The endogenomorphic depressions . . . regularly result in a sharp, unreactive, pervasive impairment of their capacity to experience pleasure or to respond affectively to the anticipation of pleasure. The key inhibition of the pleasure mechanism results in a profound lack of interest and investment in the environment' [7].

Klein, however, also recognized demoralization: 'One aspect of psychiatric illness that is frequently not clearly understood is demoralization. Demoralization is the belief in one's ineffectiveness, engendered by a severe life defeat. It is a change in self-image (the complex of attitudes and evaluations towards the self) in the direction of helplessness. Any life defeat may produce demoralization' [8].

Klein recognized that this demoralization was distinguishable from the anhedonic form of depression, yet could occur with it. Furthermore, in his understanding, it did not respond to antidepressant medication and often persisted longer than the anhedonic form of depression: 'Depression is particularly prone to produce demoralization since a feature of the pathological depressive mood is the profound conviction that one is incapable . . . Even after the pathological mood [anhedonia] has remitted so that enjoyment is possible, the ability to anticipate and plan competent activity may be severely diminished because of persistent change in self-image . . . It is a secondary, though now autonomous, cognitive residue of a past affective state' [8].

Klein also notes grief as something that can be confused with, and needs to be distinguished from, clinical depression: 'Even severe mourning can usually be simply discriminated from retarded depressions. In the mourning state, the patient is concerned about his loss and his thinking revolves around the lost object. In depression, the patient is concerned about himself and his thinking revolves about his painful depressed state' [8].

In the study by Clarke *et al.* [5] in medical inpatients, 30% of depressed persons acknowledged that their experience was 'as if they had lost something'. In other words, a bereavement-like experience was occurring in the absence of the death of a loved one. As Klein and Davis [8] have pointed out, 'loss of a valued ideal, business or career goal may precipitate analogous states'. C.M. Parkes also has applied the model of loss and bereavement to the experience of physical illness and injury [9].

It could be noted also that, although grief states share some phenomena with post-trauma syndromes – most particularly distress following a serious event, and recurrent, intrusive and distressing thoughts, memories or dreams – they are quite distinct. In normal bereavement, there is pining and longing; the person seeks out and wants to talk; the overwhelming emotion is sorrow. In post-trauma situations, the overwhelming emotion is anxiety and this is made worse with exposure to memories of the traumatic event; behaviour is avoidant [10, 11].

Change and facing adversity is a part of life, though cancer throws up special challenges, and some people cope better than others. This is about adapting to change, re-evaluating life, perhaps setting new goals, accepting the loss of things that cannot be regained, and moving forward with competence and vitality in the life ahead. Demoralization describes a failure to make this adaptation successfully, leading to hopelessness, despair and depression.

COPING

Traditionally, and as described by Lazarus and Folkman [12], coping is viewed as a transaction between the individual and the environment. Coping theory is usually couched within a cognitive framework and emphasizes cognitive appraisal in determining an individual's emotional response to stress. Primary appraizal is the person's evaluation of the personal significance of a given stressful event. This includes judgements about harm or loss, threatened harm or loss, or challenge. Secondary appraisals are the person's evaluation of the adequacy of his/her resources for coping – either personal and internal resources, or social and external resources.

Lazarus and Folkman also distinguished two types of coping behaviour: problem-focused and emotion-focused. Problem-focused coping is defined as efforts focused on the environment and the problem at hand – that is, efforts and actions to control or ameliorate the problem. In contrast, emotion-focused coping is involved more with reducing exposure to the stressor and its associated emotion – using escape and avoidance, distancing, distraction, seeking social support, and cognitive reframing. In general, a problem-solving approach is expected to lead to a favourable outcome – a solving of the problem and a reduction in anxiety. However, in acute crises, just monitoring and coping with emotions becomes a very important task. In acute medical illness, confrontational problem-focused coping is commonly employed [13]. On the other hand, acceptance-resignation emotion-focused coping is typically seen in people with chronic illness with little expectation of recovery [13, 14]. Patients under stress, indeed those who are demoralized, use a combination of all

Table 2.1   Styles of adjustment to cancer (adapted from Moorey & Greer [16]).

	View of illness	Control	Prognosis
Fighting spirit	Challenge	Some control	Good
Avoidance or denial	Minimal threat	Irrelevant	Good
Fatalism	Minor threat	No control	Uncertain - accepted with equanimity
Hopelessness-helplessness	Major threat or loss	No control	Inevitably negative
Anxious Preoccupation	Major threat	Uncertain control	Uncertain

coping mechanisms, combining confrontation with avoidance and acceptance-resignation [6].

Stroebe and Schut [15], in the 'dual process' model of coping, highlight the importance of doing both – on the one hand facing and dealing with the painful emotion, and on the other periodically taking time out from the pain of grief.

Moorey and Greer [16] have used this cognitive attributional model in understanding patients' adjustment to cancer. Three things determine a person's emotional response: (a) view of diagnosis (e.g. as a challenge or threat), (b) perception of control (some or none), and (c) view of prognosis (good or bad) (see Table 2.1). So, for instance, the helplessness-hopelessness attitude arises when the illness is seen as a major threat or loss, there is no perceived control over the illness, and the outcome is considered inevitably negative. A fighting spirit arises when the diagnosis is seen as a challenge, there is some perception of control, and the prognosis is optimistic. Our emotional reactions depend on our appraisal of the situation as much as the reality of the situation, and our sense of competency and control.

ADAPTING TO LIFE CIRCUMSTANCES – CHANGING OUR ASSUMPTIONS

In chronic or life-limiting illness, or after a loss or bereavement, a totally favourable outcome is not possible. Not all problems can be solved in the way we would like. Things are lost, not to be regained. Hopes can be dashed forever.

Changing circumstances require changing goals, ambitions and hopes. More fundamental than that, the changing circumstance may challenge the way we think about the world – for instance, as a safe and nurturing place. And it may challenge the way we think about ourselves – no longer a competent or optimistic person. Parkes describes this 'assumptive world' as 'the individual's view of reality as he [or she] believes it to be': 'It includes, for instance, the assumption ... that when I go home at night my wife will be there to greet me and that when I get up in the morning I can stand and walk about' [17].

Antonovsky [18] has used the expression 'sense of coherence' to describe a similar concept. Working within a *salutogenic* approach to health, focusing on those factors involved in a person's movement toward wellness, he describes three attitudes to the world as being key components of sense of coherence. These are *comprehensibility* (the world is structured, predictable and explicable), *manageability* (internal and external resources are available to meet the challenges) and *meaningfulness* (the demands and challenges are worthy of investment and engagement) [19]. Once developed through childhood years, sense of coherence is fairly robust in adulthood, strengthening slightly as one gets older. It determines to a large extent how one copes with adversities such as cancer.

To some extent these beliefs and perceptions – of manageability, for instance – are illusory. Indeed, most healthy adults are positively biased in their self perceptions [20], and yet cancer and other major life events do necessarily challenge these assumptions [17]. Adjusting to cancer involves a review of these very important existential issues – our view of the world, our degree of control, and the ultimate meaning of our lives, relationships and endeavours.

A REVISED MODEL OF COPING

S. Folkman [21] has proposed an adaptation to the traditional model of coping (Figure 2.1). Whereas the original model focused on distress, and on problem-solving to alleviate the problem and avoidance

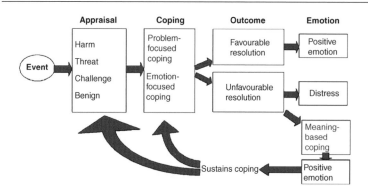

Figure 2.1   Folkman's revised model of coping (from Folkman & Greer [22]). Adapted from Folkman & Greer 2000.

behaviours when that was not possible, Folkman studied a group of people experiencing an unfavourable event outcome but who had a favourable emotion outcome – that is, were not becoming depressed. The study group were people with AIDS and their carers. From her observations, she described a third type of coping which she called meaning-based. In meaning-based coping, people: (a) used positive appraisal (see something positive in the circumstance), (b) found meaning in daily life events, (c) revised goals for the future, and (d) activated spiritual beliefs.

The use of each of these seemed to generate a sense of meaning and purpose, leading to positive emotional states [22]. What is more, the relationship between components was not linear or in one direction. A positive mood invigorated confidence, leading to more positive appraisals and more adaptive behaviours.

THE FINDING OF MEANING

There has been in recent years a considerable amount of literature in the cancer field looking at the role of meaning. Of course, the search for meaning is as old as history itself, and in the last century, its importance in human experience and flourishing has been exemplified by the writings of people such as V. Frankl. For Frankl [23], the discovery of meaning was generally gained through creative endeavour and the appreciation of beauty; but when these were unavailable, those who did well displayed their yearning for life through commitments or responsibilities beyond the present situation – sustained by values and beliefs that transcended the present circumstance. Making sense of a situation and finding some benefit from it are components of 'finding meaning' [24]. Having a 'global' sense of meaning has been shown to be an important protective factor against the development of depression and demoralization in cancer patients [25].

DEMORALIZATION AND DEPRESSION

A. Beck, a leader in the cognitive understanding of depression, described three characteristic negative cognitions of depression [26]. The 'triad', as it was called, involved thoughts of self (as worthless), the world (as hostile) and the future (as hopeless). Abramson *et al.* [27], following on the work of M. Seligman, emphasized the importance of pervasive expectancies of no control ('learned helplessness') in the development of depression. This cognitive style leads to negative beliefs about personal competence and worth, and exaggerated negative assumptions about outcomes. Depression marked by prominent hopelessness derives from situations where desired outcomes will not occur and/or adverse outcomes will occur, and where no response appears to be able to change the outcome [28]. Helplessness leads to hopelessness.

As described above, Clarke *et al.* conducted a series of studies in the medically ill, some of these qualitative [29], and others quantitative in the form of numeric taxonomy [5, 6, 30]. The results suggest the existence of (at least) three different syndromes: demoralization, anhedonic depression and grief. The demoralization which was described [31] is evidently the same thing as that described by the previously mentioned researchers, D. Klein (demoralization), S. Greer (hopelessness/helplessness) and L. Abramson (hopelessness depression). It is also a similar concept to the 'giving up-given up' complex described by G. Engel [32], occurring often as a prelude to medical illness and also characterized by hopelessness and helplessness. And finally we note the work of J. Frank, arguably the person most strongly associated with the concept, who describes demoralization as '[resulting] from persistent failure to cope with internally or externally induced stresses that the person and those close to him expect him to handle. The characteristic features . . . are feelings of impotence, isolation and despair. The person's self esteem is damaged and he feels rejected by others because of his failure to meet their expectations. Insofar as the meaning and significance of life derives from an individual's ties with persons whose values he shares, alienation may contribute to a sense of the meaninglessness of life' [33]. 'Typically [such people] are conscious of having failed to meet their own expectations or those of others, or of being unable to cope with some pressing problem. They feel powerless to change the situation for themselves and cannot extricate themselves from their predicament' [34].

A common phrase patients use that indicates the beginning of demoralization is 'I cannot cope'. At that point they are beginning to descend into demoralization, the key elements of which are helplessness, hopelessness, a subjective sense of incompetence, shame, aloneness, disconnection from others, despair and ultimately futility – seeing no purpose in going on (see Figure 2.2). Subjective incompetence is a key feature of demoralization, distinguishing it from melancholic or anhedonic depression [35]. Demoralized persons are paralysed by helplessness and not knowing what to do; melancholics are paralysed by their lack of internal drive and motivation that prevents them taking initiative even when they know what to do. Shame, guilt and diminished self esteem are also commonly recognized components of a depressive syndrome, but are only just beginning to receive attention as an important part of the cancer experience [36, 37].

Demoralization involves a loss of hope, esteem, purpose and meaning. These are state phenomena, but are closely related to their

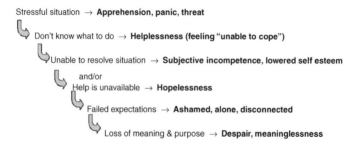

Stressful situation → **Apprehension, panic, threat**

↳ Don't know what to do → **Helplessness (feeling "unable to cope")**

 ↳ Unable to resolve situation → **Subjective incompetence, lowered self esteem**

  ↳ and/or
   Help is unavailable → **Hopelessness**

    ↳ Failed expectations → **Ashamed, alone, disconnected**

     ↳ Loss of meaning & purpose → **Despair, meaninglessness**

Figure 2.2   The process of demoralization.

trait equivalents. A strong generalized hope will preserve the meaning of life when particular hopes are quashed. A strong self esteem will maintain confidence when things get tough.

To explore this empirically, Boscaglia and Clarke [38] measured sense of coherence in 120 women with gynaecological cancer. Using sense of coherence as the dependent variable, they found that demoralization accounted for 60% of its variance. One's 'assumptive world', that is, one's beliefs about the meaning, manageability and comprehensibility of the world, do affect the way one responds to crises.

TREATMENT IMPLICATIONS

This chapter does not aim to deal with treatment considerations. Nevertheless, a short discussion will allow some of the implications of the concepts of adaptation and of demoralization for treatment to be drawn out.

J. Frank maintained that demoralization was what responded *par excellence* to psychotherapy [33]. Indeed, it was the occurrence of demoralization and the 'common features' of the various techniques that accounted for much of the effectiveness of psychotherapy [39]. This is in stark contrast to depression marked by anhedonia, which arguably does require antidepressant pharmacotherapy [40]. Grief, on the other hand, is not to be treated and cured, only assisted [41]. This taxonomy is not meant to imply that each of the three conditions occurs independently of the other. They may occur together, but their treatments are different. We should not expect, for example, to remove the sorrow of grief with medication. Furthermore, demoralization may improve if the anhedonic component of the depression is lessened with antidepressant medication, or pain attenuated with analgesia.

Frank described the 'common features' of psychotherapies to be: (a) an emotionally charged confiding therapeutic relationship, (b) an explanation for the patient's distress, (c) provision of useful information, (d) giving the patient positive expectations, (e) provision of success experiences, and (f) facilitating emotional expression [39]. These can be more or less applied to the problem of demoralization. Good information will reduce much anxiety and distress. Effective symptom control, and involving the patient in decision-making, will significantly reduce helplessness. Facilitating contact and meaningful conversations with the family will encourage authentic communication and reduce aloneness. Much of this is done by the medical and nursing staff in their usual care. For severely demoralized patients, more expert counselling is required.

CONCLUSIONS

In this chapter, I have described three different syndromes observed in cancer patients: anhedonic depression, demoralization and grief. The last two lend themselves to psychological understanding and to psychological interventions. To the extent that a person feels demoralized – that is, helpless, hopeless, alone and despairing – he/she will be helped by reducing helplessness and fear of the unknown, by conveying realistic optimism, and by being treated with dignity and respect. Specific help at reviewing goals and exploring meaning will be a task for a counsellor or psychotherapist. Sorrow about things lost, either real or imagined, needs to be supported. Often denial in facing these things needs to be gently challenged. The time of diagnosis of cancer or cancer recurrence is a stressful time, confronting very basic existential issues. Yet, many people cope well.

Understanding the normal processes of human coping and adaptation, and identifying those patients at risk because of poor internal (personality, cognitive style) or external (social) resources will assist us to recognize what is going on with the cancer patients and how to best help them.

REFERENCES

1. Cassell, E.J. (1991) *The Nature of Suffering and the Goals of Medicine*, Oxford University Press, Oxford.
2. Greer, S. and Watson, M. (1987) Mental adjustment to cancer: its measurement and prognostic importance. *Cancer Surv.*, **6,** 439–458.
3. Watson, M., Haviland, J.S., Greer, S. *et al.* (1999) Influence of psychological response on survival in breast cancer: a population based cohort study. *Lancet*, **354,** 1331–1336.

4. Jacobsen, J.C., Vanderwerker, L.C., Block, S.D. *et al.* (2006) Depression and demoralization as distinct syndromes: preliminary data from a cohort of advanced cancer patients. *Indian J. Palliat. Care*, **12**, 8–15.

5. Clarke, D.M., Mackinnon, A.J., Smith, G.C. *et al.* (2000) Dimensions of psychopathology in the medically ill: a latent trait analysis. *Psychosomatics*, **41**, 418–425.

6. Clarke, D.M., Kissane, D.W., Trauer, T. and Smith, G.C. (2005) Demoralization, anhedonia and grief in patients with severe physical illness. *World Psychiatry*, **4**, 96–105.

7. Klein, D.F. (1974) Endogenomorphic depression. *Arch. Gen. Psychiatry*, **31**, 447–454.

8. Klein, D.F. and Davis, J.M. (1969) *Diagnosis and Drug Treatment of Psychiatric Disorders*, Williams & Wilkins, Baltimore.

9. Parkes, C.M. (1972) Components of the reaction to loss of a limb, spouse or home. *J. Psychosom. Res.*, **16**, 343–349.

10. Stroebe, M., Schut, H. and Finkenauer, C. (2001) The traumatisation of grief? A conceptual framework for understanding the trauma-bereavement interface. *Israel J. Psychiatry*, **38**, 185–201.

11. Raphael, B. and Martinek, N. (1997) Assessing traumatic bereavement and posttraumatic stress disorder, in *Assessing Psychological Trauma and PTSD* (eds. J.P. Wilson and T.M. Keane), Guilford, New York, pp. 373–395.

12. Lazarus, R.S. and Folkman, S. (1984) *Stress, Appraisal, and Coping*, Springer, New York.

13. Feifel, H., Strack, S. and Nagy, V.T. (1987) Coping strategies and associated features of medical inpatients. *Psychosom. Med.*, **49**, 616–625.

14. Lipowski, Z.J. (1970) Physical illness, the individual and the coping processes. *Psychiatr. Med.*, **1**, 91–102.

15. Stroebe, M. and Schut, H. (1999) The dual process model of coping with bereavement: rationale and description. *Death Stud.*, **23**, 197–224.

16. Moorey, S. and Greer, S. (1989) *Psychological Therapy for Patients with Cancer: A New Approach*, American Psychiatric Press, Washington.

17. Parkes, C.M. (1975) What becomes of redundant world models? A contribution to the study of adaptation to change. *Br. J. Med. Psychol.*, **48**, 131–137.

18. Antonovsky, A. (1979) *Health, Stress and Coping*, Jossey-Bass, San Francisco.

19. Antonovsky, A. (1987) *Unravelling the Mystery of Health: How People Manage Stress and Stay Well*, Jossey-Bass, San Francisco.

20. Taylor, S.E. and Brown, J.D. (1988) Illusion and well-being: a social psychological perspective on mental health. *Psychol. Bull.*, **103**, 193–210.

21. Folkman, S. (1997) Positive psychological states and coping with severe stress. *Soc. Sci. Med.*, **45**, 1207–1221.

22. Folkman, S. and Greer, S. (2000) Promoting psychological wellbeing in the face of serious illness: when theory, research and practice inform each other. *Psychooncology*, **9**, 11–19.

23. Frankl, V.E. (1973) *The Doctor and the Soul: From Psychotherapy to Logotherapy*, Vintage Books, New York.

24. Davis, C.G., Nolen-Hoeksema, S. and Larson, J. (1998) Making sense of loss and benefitting from the experience: two construals of meaning. *J. Pers. Soc. Psychol.*, **75**, 561–574.

25. Vehling, S., Lehman, C., Oechsle, K. *et al.* (2010) Global meaning and meaning-related life attitudes: exploring their role in predicting depression, anxiety, and demoralization in cancer patients. *Support. Care Cancer* (in press).

26. Beck, A.T. (1987) Cognitive models of depression. *J. Cogn. Psychother.*, **1**, 5–37.

27. Abramson, L.Y., Metalsky, G.I. and Allow, L.B. (1989) Hopelessness depression: a theory based subtype of depression. *Psychol. Rev.*, **96**, 358–372.

28. Abramson, L.Y., Metalsky, G.I. and Alloy, L.B. (1993) Hopelessness, in *Symptoms of Depression* (ed. C.G. Costello), John Wiley, New York, pp. 85–112.

29. Clarke, D.M., Cook, K.E., Coleman, K.J. and Smith, G.C. (2006) A qualitative examination of the experience of 'depression' in hospitalized medically ill patients. *Psychopathology*, **39**, 303–312.

30. Clarke, D.M., Smith, G.C., Dowe, D.L. and McKenzie, D.P. (2003) An empirically derived taxonomy of common distress syndromes in the medically ill. *J. Psychosom. Res.*, **54**, 323–330.

31. Clarke, D.M. and Kissane, D.W. (2002) Demoralization: its phenomenology and importance. *Aust. N. Z. J. Psychiatry*, **6**, 733–742.

32. Engel, G.L. (1967) A psychological setting of somatic disease: the Giving Up-Given Up complex. *Proc. R. Soc. Med.*, **60**, 553–555.

33. Frank, J.D. (1974) Psychotherapy: the restoration of morale. *Am. J. Psychiatry*, **131**, 271–274.

34. Frank, J.D. and Frank, J.B. (1991) *Persuasion and Healing: A Comparative Study of Psychotherapy*, 3rd edn, Johns Hopkins University Press, Baltimore.

35. de Figueiredo, J.M. (1993) Depression and demoralization: phenomen-ologic differences and research perspectives. *Compr. Psychiatry*, **34,** 308–311.
36. Chapple, A., Zeibland, S. and McPherson, A. (2004) Stigma, shame and blame experienced by patients with lung cancer: qualitative study. *BMJ*, **328,** 1470.
37. LoConte, N.K., Else-Quest, N.M., Eickhoff, J. *et al.* (2008) Assessment of guilt and shame in patients with non-small-cell lung cancer compared with patients with breast and prostate cancer. *Clin. Lung Cancer*, **9,** 171–178.
38. Boscaglia, N. and Clarke, D.M. (2007) Sense of Coherence as a protective factor for demoralization in women with a recent diagnosis of gynaecological cancer. *Psychooncology*, **16,** 189–195.
39. Frank, J.D. (1972) The common features of psychotherapy. *Aust. N. Z. J. Psychiatry*, **6,** 34–40.
40. Snaith, R.P. (1987) The concepts of mild depression. *Br. J. Psychiatry*, **150,** 387–393.
41. Worden, J.W. (2002) *Grief Counselling and Grief Therapy: A Handbook for the Mental Health Practitioner*, 3rd edn, Springer, New York.

CHAPTER 3

Biology of Depression and Cytokines in Cancer

**Dominique L. Musselman, Andrew H. Miller,
Erica B. Royster and Marcia D. McNutt**
*Laboratory of Neuropsychopharmacology, Department of Psychiatry and
Behavioral Sciences, Emory University School of Medicine,
Atlanta, GA, USA*

Buttressing the identification of grief, demoralization, hopelessness and styles of psychological coping of the cancer patient are vital, ongoing scientific developments that flow from an increased understanding of the interplay amongst the immune system, endocrine system, and brain. The evolving understanding of this interplay between the neurobiology of the stress response and neuroimmune function, immunoinflammatory pathways associated with cancer and its treatment, and resulting neurobehavioural symptoms, represent a quintessential 'mind-body' interface (Figure 3.1). This rapidly accumulating body of neurobiologic knowledge has catalyzed fundamental changes in how we conceptualize depressive symptoms and has important implications regarding the treatment, and even prevention, of depressive symptoms in patients afflicted with cancer.

THE BIOLOGY OF DEPRESSION

Within a biopsychosocial model of the aetiology of depression, the biological contribution could be best understood as a preexisting

Depression and Cancer   Edited by David W. Kissane, Mario Maj and Norman Sartorius
© 2011 John Wiley & Sons, Ltd

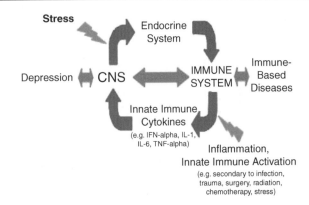

Figure 3.1 The interplay between the neurobiology of the stress response, neuroimmune function, immunoinflammatory pathways associated with cancer and its treatment, and depression.

vulnerability, which is activated by a stressful event such as cancer and its treatment. This biological vulnerability would be genetically determined [1] and then lead to an interaction between nature and nurture [2]. One such example is given by the serotonin transporter (5-HTT) gene. Variation in the 5-HTT gene affects the prospect that a patient dealing with stress will go on to experience depression, which appears more likely in those with one or two short alleles of the gene [1]. An important Swedish twin study estimated the heritability of depression – the degree to which individual differences in occurrence are associated with genetic differences – to be approximately 40% for women and 30% for men [3].

At a physiological level, this genetic perspective has been translated into the monoamine hypothesis of depression. This construct recognizes that most antidepressant medications increase the levels of one or more of the monoamine neurotransmitters – serotonin, noradrenaline and dopamine – in the synaptic cleft between cerebral neurons. Such medications may directly impact these neurotransmitter receptors. One contemporary account of the monoamine hypothesis proposes that a deficiency of certain neurotransmitters is responsible for the phenomenology of depression: thus a decrease in noradrenaline may be associated with loss of alertness, attention, energy and interest in life; a reduction in serotonin to anxiety, obsessions and compulsions; and a decrease in dopamine to loss of motivation, pleasure and reward [4].

Depression has long been recognized to be influenced by an overactive hypothalamic-pituitary-adrenal (HPA) axis, as occurs in response to stress. Elevated cortisol, as might occur with enlargement of the pituitary and adrenal glands, has been associated with depression. Oversecretion of corticotropin-releasing hormone (CRH) from the hypothalamus drives this, and has been implicated in both cognitive and arousal symptoms of depression [5]. At the gonadal level, oestrogen has also been associated with depression with onset after puberty, childbirth and menopause, when oestrogen levels fluctuate most widely [6].

Magnetic resonance imaging (MRI) of the brains of patients with depression has identified differences in both structure and function compared to non-depressed subjects. Although some inconsistency exists, meta-analyses have confirmed smaller hippocampal volumes [7]. This loss of hippocampal neurons correlates with impaired memory and dysthymic mood. Drugs that increase serotonin levels in the brain may stimulate neurogenesis and increase the total mass of the hippocampus. This then helps to restore mood and memory [8].

Similar relationships have been noted between depression and the anterior cingulate cortex in the modulation of emotional behaviour [9]. One of the neurotrophins responsible for neurogenesis here is the brain-derived neurotrophic factor (BDNF). Meta-analyses show the level of BDNF in the serum of depressed subjects to be reduced threefold [10]. Antidepressant treatment increases the blood level of BDNF. Although decreased serum BDNF is found in other mental disorders, such as schizophrenia, there is considerable interest about its relationship to depression and the action of antidepressants [10].

Depression has also been associated with immune mechanisms (understandably switched on by cancers) and the biological molecules involved in these processes termed cytokines. In many ways, the phenomenology of depression is not unlike the illness experience when the body is fighting an infection [11]. Elevated levels of circulating cytokines have been associated with depression and may explain some of the variation in depression seen in different tumours [12].

THE MORBID OUTCOME OF DEPRESSION IN CANCER PATIENTS

A number of studies have suggested that depression predisposes patients to poorer survival after they develop cancer, including women with breast cancer and men and women with lung cancer, even after controlling for prognostic factors, such as age, nicotine use, tumour grade and cancer stage [13–16]. In a study of 871 cancer patients, those with a history of depressive symptoms were found to have a 2.6 times increased risk of dying from their cancer within the first 19 months following diagnosis [17]. In another study of 103 cancer patients, a depressive coping style correlated with decreased survival time, even when other biomedical risk factors such as tumour grade and histological classification were taken into account [18]. In addition to potential direct effects on survival, depression is known to decrease compliance with therapy, increase length of hospital stay, diminish quality of life, and limit the ability to care for oneself [19–22].

Depression that develops in response to medical treatment may impact therapeutic efficacy and, by extension, decrease quality of life and survival. For example, patients who developed major depression while receiving interferon (IFN)-alpha for malignant melanoma were significantly less likely to remain on treatment than were patients without depression (5% versus 35%) [23]. Similarly, patients who became depressed following stem cell transplant were found to have a three times increased risk of dying between 6 to 12 months after the procedure, after adjusting for other prognostic factors [11]. Thus, the increased mortality of cancer patients with depression may be due, at least in part, to their diminished ability to care for themselves and/or premature discontinuation of cancer therapy [24].

INFLAMMATORY MECHANISMS AND DEVELOPMENT OF NEUROBEHAVIOURAL SYMPTOMS IN CANCER PATIENTS

A rich database substantiates the capacity of cytokines – including the pro-inflammatory cytokines tumour necrosis factor (TNF)-alpha, interleukin (IL)-1 and IL-6 – to induce a syndrome of sickness behaviour, which shares many features with major depression [25–27]. Sickness behaviour is typically associated with the behavioural changes seen in humans and laboratory animals suffering from microbial infections. It includes anhedonia, cognitive dysfunction, anxiety/irritability, psychomotor slowing, anergia/fatigue, anorexia, sleep alterations and increased sensitivity to pain [28]. Relevant to its mediation by cytokines, sickness behaviour can be reliably reproduced by administration of cytokines in isolation or by administering agents (e.g. endotoxin or lipopolysaccharide) that induce the inflammatory cytokine cascade (TNF-alpha to IL-1 to IL-6) [25].

Although cytokines are too large to freely pass through the blood brain barrier, several pathways by which cytokine signals can access the brain have been elucidated. Some of these include passage of cytokines through leaky regions in the blood-brain barrier and active transport and transmission of cytokine signals via afferent nerve fibres (e.g. vagus) [11, 26–28]. Recent data also indicate that activated immune cells (macrophages) can directly pass through the blood-brain barrier and enter the brain parenchyma [29]. Within the brain, a cytokine network has been described, consisting of cell types (glia/neurons) that can both produce cytokines and receive their signals via relevant receptors [27, 30].

Several studies suggest that cytokines may be involved in depression in both medically healthy and medically ill patients [11, 31–33], including patients with cancer (Table 3.1). Research has revealed that pro-inflammatory cytokines are elevated in cancer patients with depression and correlate with symptoms of sickness behaviour. For example, plasma concentrations of IL-6 were significantly increased in patients with cancer and depression as well as in depressed control subjects [23]. In other studies, both IL-1 and IL-6 significantly correlated with fatigue in cancer patients undergoing treatment with radiation and/or chemotherapy [34–36]. At high risk for behavioural alterations may also be those patients whose neoplastic cells produce cytokines and/or aggressive inflammatory reactions, or those individuals receiving cancer treatments involving extensive tissue damage or destruction, leading to significant immune activation/inflammation and release of pro-inflammatory cytokines (e.g. certain surgeries or radiation).

Table 3.1 Cytokines and their soluble receptors implicated in cancer

Cytokines and their receptors	Role
Interleukin-1, IL-1 [40]	Directly produced by cancer cells; can promote tumour growth and metastasis
Interleukin-1 receptor antagonist, IL-1RA [40]	A protein which binds to same receptor on the cell surface as IL-1 (IL-1R) and thus prevents IL-1 from sending a signal to that cell
Interleukin-6, IL-6 [41]	Both a pro-inflammatory and anti-inflammatory cytokine that mediates fever and the acute phase response; more IL-6 appears in blood of metastatic cancer patients
Soluble interleukin-6 receptor, sIL-6R [41]	Mediates differentiation and survival of neuronal cells; acts as IL-6 agonist by inducing cellular responses
Tumour necrosis factor-alpha, TNF-alpha [42]	Regulates immune cells by inducing cell death and inflammation, and inhibiting viral replication and cancer cell transformation from tumours
Soluble tumour necrosis receptor 2, sTNFR2 [43]	Binds to TNF and is found only in cells in immune system; tumour cells increase concentration in patients with cancer
C-reactive protein, CRP [44]	Levels rise in response to inflammation and higher concentrations are found in cancer patients; CRP level is a potential predictor of increased cancer risk

Based on these findings (albeit relatively limited to date), cytokine effects on behaviour may be most apparent in patients undergoing cytokine therapies (i.e. IL-2 or IFN-alpha), which induce the release of pro-inflammatory cytokines, such as IL-6 and TNF-alpha [31, 37–39], which in turn have been implicated in mood regulation. Thus, the immunotherapies utilizing the innate immune system cytokine IFN-alpha and the T-cell cytokine IL-2 have become model systems in which to explore not only how cytokines influence the brain and behaviour, but also which treatment strategies might be appropriate for addressing those mechanisms.

IFN-alpha is a potentially effective therapy for patients with metastatic melanoma at high risk for recurrence. However, during the initial 12 weeks of administration, severe depression or neurotoxicity has been shown to necessitate discontinuation of IFN-alpha in approximately one-third of individuals with malignant melanoma [16]. The debilitating effects of IFN-alpha have largely contributed to the recent clinical practice of truncating the year-long IFN-alpha treatment to just one month of intravenous therapy.

We examined the incidence of major depression in patients with malignant melanoma (n = 40) receiving high dose IFN-alpha therapy, randomly arranged to either preventive paroxetine treatment or placebo [19]. Of the 20 placebo-treated patients, nine (45%) developed symptoms sufficient for a diagnosis of major depression (relative risk, 0.24; 95% CI 0.08–0.93) (Figure 3.2). In addition, severe depression or neurotoxicity necessitated discontinuation of IFN-alpha prior to 12 weeks in 7 patients (35%) in the placebo group (relative risk, 0.14; 95% CI 0.05–0.85).

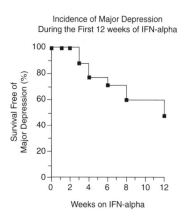

Figure 3.2 Incidence of major depression in patients with malignant melanoma receiving high dose interferon-alpha therapy (from Musselman *et al.* [19], reproduced with permission).

IMMUNE CONTRIBUTIONS TO NEUROBEHAVIOURAL SYMPTOMS IN PATIENTS WITH CANCER

In terms of mood regulation, there are at least four pathways by which cytokines may cause depression/sickness behaviour.

First, cytokines have been shown to have potent stimulatory effects on the HPA axis, in large part through activation of CRH [45, 46]. CRH has behavioural effects in animals that are similar to those seen in patients suffering from depression/sickness behaviour, including alterations in activity, appetite and sleep [47]. Moreover, as previously noted, patients with depression have been found to exhibit evidence of increased CRH activity [48, 49]. A 41-amino-acid peptide, CRH is considered one of the primary central nervous system 'stress hormones', as it coordinates immune, autonomic, endocrine and behavioural responses to stress. Within the brain, CRH is located in neurons both within and outside of the hypothalamus. Within the paraventricular nucleus of the hypothalamus, CRH-containing neurons project to the median eminence [50] and induce secretion of adrenocorticotropic hormone (ACTH) and beta-endorphin from the anterior pituitary [51]. In turn, ACTH stimulates cortisol secretion from the adrenal cortex [52]. In order to study the relationship between IFN-alpha-induced depression and HPA axis function, in the above noted study (Figure 3.2), a subset (n = 14) of the 20 placebo-treated patients with malignant melanoma receiving IFN-alpha therapy had plasma samples drawn just prior to, and then 1, 2 and 3 hours following, IFN-alpha administration. Samples were drawn again at week 2, 4, 8 and 12 of IFN-alpha therapy. Over the 12 weeks of therapy, 7 of the 14 patients developed major depression [53]. ACTH and cortisol responses, but not IL-6 responses, to the initial administration of IFN-alpha were significantly higher in the seven patients who subsequently developed major depression than in those who did not (Figure 3.3). No differences in hormonal or cytokine responses were found between these two groups *during* IFN-alpha administration. ACTH and cortisol responses to the initial injection of IFN-alpha were also significantly associated with depressive, anxious and cognitive symptoms at week 8 of IFN-alpha therapy (Table 3.2). No such correlations were found with neurovegetative (e.g. fatigue, anorexia, sleep disturbance) or somatic (e.g. pain, gastrointestinal distress)

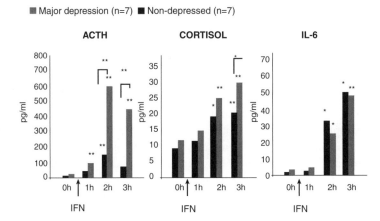

Figure 3.3 Adrenocorticotropic hormone (ACTH), cortisol and interleukin-6 (IL-6) responses to first injection of interferon-alpha (IFN-alpha) is greater in patients who later develop major depression (from Capuron *et al.* [53], reproduced with permission).

Table 3.2 Correlation between adrenocorticotropic hormone (ACTH) and cortisol responses after initial dose of interferon-alpha and depressive, anxiety and cognitive symptoms eight weeks later (from Capuron *et al.* [53], reproduced with permission)

Symptom dimension	ACTH (r)	Cortisol (r)
Depression	.699**	.534*
Anxiety	.704**	.520*
Cognitive dysfunction	.656*	.622**
Neurovegetative	.345	.400
Somatic	.293	.236

*p < 0.05
**p < 0.01

symptoms. Interestingly, mood and cognitive changes during IFN-alpha therapy were most responsive to treatment with paroxetine, suggesting that stress reactivity and CRH may be more relevant to vulnerability to cytokine-induced depression and its treatment with antidepressants than other aspects of sickness such as fatigue, anorexia and pain [23].

Second, a number of cytokines (especially IL-1, IL-6, TNF-alpha, IFN-alpha and IL-2) have been shown to alter the metabolism of noradrenaline, serotonin and dopamine, all of which have been implicated in the pathophysiology of mood disorders [56]. Cytokines, including IFN-alpha, have been shown to reduce serum concentrations of L-tryptophan, likely secondary to changes in dietary intake (due to anorexia) and the induction of the enzyme indolamine 2,3 dioxygenase, which breaks down tryptophan into kynurenine [11, 54, 56, 58]. Tryptophan is the primary precursor of serotonin, and depletion of tryptophan has been associated with the precipitation of mood disturbances in vulnerable patients [59]. Early studies revealed that the development of depressive symptoms during IFN-alpha therapy was associated with diminished peripheral blood concentrations of tryptophan [55, 60] (Table 3.2). More recent data, however, indicate that the generation of kynurenine, which is then converted to quinolinic acid and kynurenic acid in the brain, may be more relevant to mood changes than tryptophan [61, 62]. Studies in laboratory animals demonstrate that injection of kynurenine alone can induce depressive symptoms in rodents [60]. In humans, while no changes in cerebrospinal fluid (CSF) tryptophan were found in IFN-alpha-treated patients, significant increases in kynurenine, quinolinic acid and kynurenic acid were noted [61]. Higher CSF concentrations of kynurenine and quinolinic acid were correlated with higher depression scores [61].

Another mechanism by which IFN-alpha may influence serotonin metabolism is through the induction of mitogen activated protein kinase (MAPK) signalling pathways, including p38. IFN-alpha, as well as other innate immune cytokines, are potent inducers of p38 MAPK, and activation of p38 MAPK has been shown to upregulate both the expression and function of 5-HTT [63, 64]. Interestingly, enhanced 5-HTT function has been associated with seasonal affective disorder [65]. In addition, in rhesus monkeys exposed to maternal abuse and rejection as infants, our group has found significant correlations between activation of p38 in peripheral blood mononuclear cells and number of maternal rejections as infants, as well as decreases in CSF concentrations of the serotonin metabolite 5-hydroxyindoleacetic acid (5-HIAA) [66]. Of note, decreased CSF 5-HIAA concentrations have been associated with increased anxiety-like behaviour in these animals [67]. These data suggest that cytokines can inflict a 'double hit' on serotonin availability through effects on synthesis and reuptake of serotonin, both potentially contributing to reduced synaptic serotonin [68].

Data from our laboratory and others support the notion that IFN-alpha, as well as other innate immune cytokines, may also profoundly alter dopamine metabolism and the function of basal ganglia circuits, thereby contributing to cytokine-induced neurovegetative symptoms, including fatigue, psychomotor slowing, and sleep disturbances [69–75]. Dopamine in the basal ganglia is known to play an important role in the regulation of multiple behaviours, including mood, motivation/reward (hedonia), motor activity, sleep/wake cycles (arousal) and cognition [76–80].

Studies of rhesus monkeys administered with IFN-alpha have revealed that development of huddling behaviour (a behavioural equivalent of depression) in vulnerable animals is associated with significant decreases in CSF concentrations of the dopamine metabolite homovanillic acid (HVA). These results are consistent with experiments in mice that have shown that treatment with IFN-alpha for up to five days significantly decreases dopamine and its metabolite 3,4-dihydroxyphenylacetic acid (DOPAC) in whole brain homogenates [74]. These dopamine changes were associated with reduced motor activity (which is also consistent with the motor slowing and fatigue exhibited in IFN-alpha-treated patients). As shown in Figure 3.4, using a longitudinal design and positron emission tomography, we recently examined regional brain glucose metabolism before and after four weeks of intravenous IFN-alpha therapy in patients with malignant melanoma. In 12 patients with malignant melanoma devoid of metastatic disease or pre-existing behavioural alterations, whole-brain glucose metabolism was estimated by

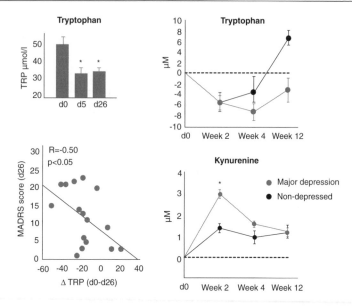

Figure 3.4 Changes in tryptophan and kynurenine in antidepressant-free patients who developed major depression compared with antidepressant-free patients who remained free of depression during IFN-α therapy (from Capuron *et al.* [54, 55], reproduced with permission). *p < 0.01.

fluorine-18-labelled fluorodeoxyglucose uptake while subjects were at rest. Significant correlations were discovered between changes (delta) in regional cerebral glucose metabolism (rCMRGLc) in the left putamen and left nucleus accumbens (relative to baseline) and changes (delta) in 'energy' subscale scores as measured by the Visual Analogue Scale of Fatigue (VAS-F) during IFN-alpha therapy ($R = -0.622$, p = 0.03 and $R = -0.669$, p = 0.02, respectively). Self-reported fatigue also correlated with increased glucose metabolism in the cerebellum. These data indicate that IFN-alpha, as well as other cytokines of the innate immune response, may target basal ganglia nuclei [81]. The increased basal ganglia resting state glucose metabolism of IFN-alpha-treated patients likely reflects altered dopaminergic activity (Figure 3.5). Increased basal ganglia metabolism has been repeatedly documented in patients with Parkinson's disease. Interestingly, treatment with levodopa or other pharmaco-

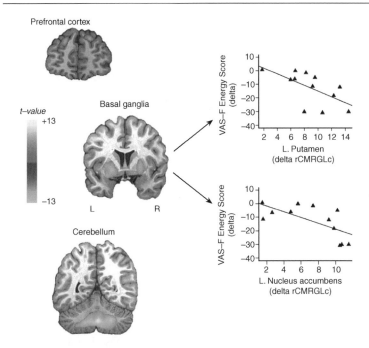

Figure 3.5 Increased metabolic activity in left basal ganglia nuclei is associated with self-reported decrease in energy during IFN-alpha therapy (from Capuron *et al.* [81], reproduced with permission).

logic agents that increase dopamine release (e.g. stimulants) have improved fatigue in patients with basal ganglia disorders as well as in IFN-alpha-treated patients [82]. Taken together, these findings suggest that changes in basal ganglia activity during IFN-alpha therapy may be related to altered dopamine neurotransmission and, in turn, play a role in the pathophysiology of IFN-alpha-induced fatigue symptoms.

Interestingly, certain of the mechanisms whereby IFN-alpha can perturb serotonin metabolism overlap with those described above which influence dopamine. For example, intrastriatal administration of kynurenic acid dramatically reduces extracellular dopamine in rat striatum [62, 83]. Interferon-alpha and other innate immune cytokines may also influence dopamine metabolism through activation of MAPK signalling pathways.

Finally, a fourth potential pathway by which pro-inflammatory cytokines may induce alterations of mood is the pituitary-thyroid axis. Pro-inflammatory cytokines have been associated with the euthyroid sick syndrome (ESS), that is characterized by normal TSH and T4 levels and reduced T3 levels in the early stages, and by normal TSH and reduced T3 and T4 in the later stages [84]. The mechanism by which ESS occurs is believed to involve both direct effects of cytokines on thyroid gland function as well as inhibition of the metabolic enzymes (5′-deiodination) that convert peripheral T4 to T3 (the more biologically active form of thyroid hormone), especially in the liver [84].

As with the pro-inflammatory cytokines, IL-2 has also been shown to influence both neuroendocrine and monoamine function. For example, IL-2 administration stimulates the release of CRH from the amygdala and hypothalamus, an effect that appears to be mediated in part by nitric oxide [85]. Repeated administration of IL-2 to mice has been found to increase the turnover of noradrenaline within the median eminence and hippocampus, alter serotonin levels in the hippocampus and prefrontal cortex, and reduce dopamine turnover in the caudate and substantia nigra [86]. All of these brain regions are involved in symptoms relevant to depression. In contrast to pro-inflammatory cytokines, IL-2 administered over five days has been shown to stimulate the pituitary-thyroid axis in patients with HIV infection [87]. Free thyroxine levels were elevated to hyperthyroid levels in these IL-2 treated patients. Relevant to cytokine-induced behavioural changes, even subtle alterations in thyroid hormone availability (both hyper- and hypothyroidism) are known to be associated with mood disorders [88].

CYTOKINES AND THE INDUCTION OF DISTINCT NEUROBEHAVIOURAL SYNDROMES

Based on clinical and animal studies, our group has proposed that IFN-alpha induces distinct neurobehavioural syndromes, which differ in time of onset as well as treatment responsiveness. Using dimensional analyses of the incidence of neurobehavioural symptoms during the first three months of IFN-alpha treatment of patients with malignant melanoma, a complex of neurovegetative symptoms including anorexia, fatigue, altered sleep and psychomotor retardation developed within two weeks of IFN-alpha therapy in a large proportion of patients. In contrast, symptoms of depressed mood, anxiety and irritability appeared later during IFN-alpha treatment. Symptoms of depression and anxiety were more responsive to treatment with paroxetine than symptoms of fatigue, psychomotor slowing, altered sleep, and anorexia. Consistent with these findings in IFN-alpha-treated patients are data showing the differential clustering of mood vs. neurovegetative symptoms in patients with cancer as well as the lack of antidepressant responsiveness of cancer-related fatigue [89, 90]. The mood/anxiety and neurovegetative syndromes appear to be mediated by different pathophysiological mechanisms, that is CRH sensitivity and perturbations of serotonin metabolism vs. dopamine pathways, respectively [91].

As discussed above, we randomly assigned 40 patients with malignant melanoma to either paroxetine or placebo two weeks prior to their initiating IFN-alpha [19]. Severe depression or neurotoxicity necessitated discontinuation of IFN-alpha prior to 12 weeks in one patient (5%) in the paroxetine group versus 7 patients (35%) in the placebo group (relative risk, 0.14; 95% CI 0.05–0.85). Paroxetine treatment significantly reduced rating scale scores of depression ($p < 0.001$), anxiety ($p < 0.001$) and neurotoxicity ($p < 0.001$) over the course of the study; neurovegetative symptoms of fatigue and anorexia did not improve (Figure 3.6). These data are consistent with the study by Morrow *et al.* [92], who found that treatment with paroxetine significantly reduced depression but not fatigue in a large sample of patients with cancer undergoing chemotherapy. This evidence suggests that pretreatment with paroxetine represents an effective strategy for minimizing IFN-alpha-induced mood symptoms and improving treatment adherence (Figure 3.7). However, different treatment strategies appear to be required to target the neurovegetative symptoms induced by this (and other) cytokine therapy.

Investigations are also ongoing to understand the differential mechanisms of symptom development in patients receiving the T-cell cytokine IL-2 [93]. The few studies that have focused on the behavioural and cognitive effects of IL-2 treatment reveal a high incidence

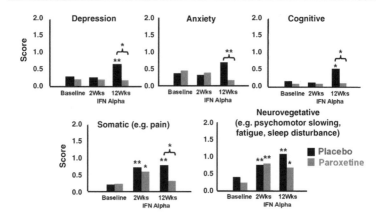

Figure 3.6 Depressive, anxious, cognitive, neurovegetative and somatic symptoms in patients treated with placebo (n = 20) or paroxetine (n = 18) during interferon-alpha. *p < 0.05; **p < 0.01. Asterisks at the top of bars indicate significant within-group differences vs. baseline. Brackets indicate inter-group differences for that time point (from Ref. [89], reproduced with permission).

of depressive symptoms and memory disturbances, but also a susceptibility of these patients to develop psychosis and/or delirium [94].

TREATMENT IMPLICATIONS

Important avenues for future research include psychotherapeutic and behavioural interventions in patients with cancer. These interventions can potentially ameliorate cytokine-related neurobehavioural comorbidity by reducing stress and inflammatory responses of the neuroendocrine system, which will directly affect the neuroendocrine-immune interaction [95]. Cognitive-behavioural techniques and interventions focusing on stress reduction and mindfulness seem to be essential, as they have been found to reduce psychological distress in breast cancer patients [96]. Furthermore, cognitive-behavioural therapy has shown to improve fatigue in over half of the cancer survivors in a recent randomized controlled trial [97]. The programme focused on sleep (e.g. sleep-wake habits and social rhythms), physical activity (e.g. aerobic exercise), coping and social

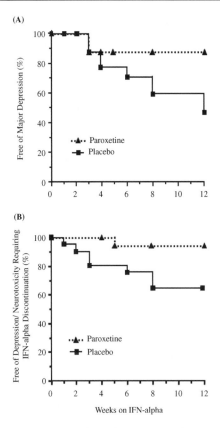

Figure 3.7 Paroxetine protects from depression and neurotoxicity necessitating treatment withdrawal when treatment with interferon-alpha is given (from Musselman *et al.* [19], reproduced with permission).

support, and these strategies seem to be relevant in the regulation of the inflammatory response in the neuroendocrine system [98–108]. Irwin *et al.* [109] found that sleep quality, sleep onset, and sleep maintenance in adults with insomnia improved with behavioural treatments, yet there is little evidence to show improvement in cancer patients [110, 111] due to lack of control group and small sample size [112, 113]. Certainly, future investigations of these interventions for patients with cancer would be bolstered by assessments of their impact on cortisol rhythms, inflammatory mediators, and neurobehavioural symptom complexes.

Pharmacologic agents that target specific pathways may alleviate specific neurobehavioural symptom domains induced by inflammation. CRH, which is stimulated by inflammatory cytokines, is an obvious target [95]. There is some preliminary indication that CRH antagonists may be effective in treating depression in medically healthy individuals [114]. Furthermore, agents that enhance glucocorticoid-mediated negative feedback of CRH pathways (e.g. phosphodiesterase type IV inhibitors), through facilitation of glucocorticoid receptor function, may decrease cytokine-induced mood and anxiety symptoms. These compounds may have the additional advantage of inhibiting immunoinflammatory pathways [115].

Other pharmacologic options currently available do selectively target monoamine neurotransmitter pathways and may ameliorate certain cytokine-induced neurobehavioural symptoms, that is, serotonergic drugs for mood/anxiety symptoms, or dopaminergic drugs for fatigue and psychomotor slowing. Paroxetine has been shown to be effective in reducing depression in two double-blind, placebo-controlled trials in cancer patients, but was ineffective in improving fatigue [89, 92]. An obvious candidate drug which needs to be tested in a large-scale, randomized, placebo-controlled, clinical trial for treatment of cancer-related fatigue is methylphenidate [116], which has been shown to treat fatigue and improve neuropsychological functioning in patients with tumour-related organic brain dysfunction [117, 118].

As research sheds further light upon the relationship between inflammatory markers and neurobehavioural symptoms in cancer patients, cytokine antagonists, anti-inflammatory agents, and medications that disrupt cytokine signalling pathways may offer other pharmacologic options. Such agents which target upstream elements of the NF-kB and p38 pathways [119, 120] are currently being studied for their antineoplastic effectiveness. Thus, investigators will have the opportunity to examine whether these agents diminish neurobehavioural morbidity in cancer patients. For example, one study has documented that the TNF-alpha inhibitor etanercept improved tolerability of chemotherapy (and reduced fatigue) in patients with advanced cancer [121].

Chronobiotic agents, such as light therapy or melatonin receptor agonists, might synchronize the circadian rhythms of cancer patients to their environment, similar to the treatment of sleep disturbances caused by shift work or long-distance travel. Chronobiotic treatment might potentially restore rhythmicity of neuroendocrine systems, alleviate inflammation, and improve effectiveness of antineoplastic therapy [122,123].

CONCLUSIONS

In the past, the increased prevalence of depression in cancer patients has been conceptualized as an emotional response to extreme stress, including overwhelming emotional loss, physical pain, and often social isolation. Investigations of cancer patients suffering from major depression revealed that neuroendocrine perturbations of these individuals (i.e. HPA axis hyperactivity) are likely due to CRH hypersecretion associated with depression and/or the potent stimulation of pro-inflammatory cytokines in response to infection, tumour progression, or antineoplastic interventions. During the past two decades, characterization of cytokine-induced mood/anxiety and neurovegetative sickness behaviour symptoms in humans has proceeded in concert with an increasing understanding of the associated alterations of immunoinflammatory pathways and monoamine neurotransmitters, especially evident in individuals receiving immunotherapies. As certain cytokine-induced symptoms, that is mood and anxiety symptoms, improve with antidepressant treatment, the quest has begun for effective interventions to relieve cytokine-induced fatigue, sleep and other neurovegetative symptoms.

A continuing impetus for the fourth decade of neurobehavioural-neuroendocrine-immune research will be to understand the neurobiology of neurobehavioural symptoms induced by cytokines in patients with cancer and other serious medical disorders, and to aggressively treat them.

REFERENCES

1. Caspi, A., Sugden, K., Moffitt, T.E. *et al.* (2003) Influence of life stress on depression: moderation by a polymorphism in the 5-HTT gene. *Science*, **301**, 386–389.

2. Haeffel, D.J., Getchell, M., Koposov, R.A. *et al.* (2008) Association between polymorphisms in the dopamine transporter gene and depression. Evidence for a gene-environment interaction in a sample of juvenile detainees. *Psychol. Sci.*, **19**, 62–69.

3. Kendler, K.S., Gatz, M., Gardner, C.O. and Pedersen, N.L. (2006) A Swedish national twin study of lifetime major depression. *Am. J. Psychiatry*, **163**, 109–114.

4. Nutt, D.J. (2008) Relationship of neurotransmitters to the symptoms of major depressive disorder. *J. Clin. Psychiatry*, **69** (Suppl. E1), 4–7.

5. Monteleone, P. (2001) Endocrine disturbances and psychiatric disorders. *Curr. Opin. Psychiatry*, **14**, 605–610.

6. Cutter, W.J., Norbury, R. and Murphy, D.G. (2003) Oestrogen, brain function, and neuropsychiatric disorders. *J. Neurol. Neurosurg. Psychiatry*, **74**, 837–840.

7. Videbech, P. and Ravnkilde, B. (2004) Hippocampal volume and depression: a meta-analysis of MRI studies. *Am. J. Psychiatry*, **161**, 1957–1966.

8. Sheline, Y.I., Gado, M.H. and Kraemer, H.C. (2003) Untreated depression and hippocampal volume loss. *Am. J. Psychiatry*, **160**, 1516–1518.

9. Drevets, W.C., Savitz, J. and Trimble, M. (2008) The subgenual anterior cingulate cortex in mood disorders. *CNS Spect.*, **13**, 663–681.

10. Sen, S., Duman, R. and Sanacora, G. (2008) Serum BDNF, depression and anti-depressant medications: meta-analyses and implications. *Biol. Psychiatry*, **64**, 527–532.

11. Dantzer, R., O'Connor, J.C., Freund, G.G. *et al.* (2008) From inflammation to sickness and depression: when the immune system subjugates the brain. *Nat. Rev. Neurosci.*, **9**, 46–56.

12. Massie, M.J. (2004) Prevalence of depression in patients with cancer. *J. Natl. Cancer Inst. Monogr.*, **32**, 57–71.

13. Watson, M., Haviland, J.S., Greer, S. *et al.* (1999) Influence of psychological response on survival in breast cancer: a population-based cohort study. *Lancet*, **354**, 1331–1336.

14. Buccheri, G. (1998) Depressive reactions to lung cancer are common and often followed by a poor outcome. *Eur. Respir. J.*, **11**, 173–178.

15. Faller, H., Bulzebruck, H., Drings, P. and Lang, H. (1999) Coping, distress, and survival among patients with lung cancer. *Arch. Gen. Psychiatry*, **56**, 756–762.

16. Herrmann, C., Brand-Driehorst, S., Kaminsky, B. *et al.* (1998) Diagnostic groups and depressed mood as predictors of 22-month mortality in medical inpatients. *Psychosom. Med.*, **60**, 570–577.

17. Stoudemire, A. and Thompson, T.L. 2nd (1983) Medication noncompliance: systematic approaches to evaluation and intervention. *Gen. Hosp. Psychiatry*, **5**, 233–239.
18. Pelletier, G., Verhoef, M.J., Khatri, N. and Hagan, N. (2002) Quality of life in brain tumor patients: the relative contributions of depression, fatigue, emotional distress, and existential issues. *J. Neurooncol.*, **57**, 41–49.
19. Musselman, D.L., Lawson, D.H., Gumnick, J.F. *et al.* (2001) Paroxetine for the prevention of depression induced by high-dose interferon alfa. *N. Engl. J. Med.*, **344**, 961–966.
20. DiMatteo, M.R., Lepper, H.S. and Croghan, T.W. (2000) Depression is a risk factor for noncompliance with medical treatment: meta-analysis of the effects of anxiety and depression on patient adherence. *Arch. Int. Med.*, **160**, 2101–2107.
21. Loberiza, F.R.J., Rizzo, J.D., Bredeson, C.N. *et al.* (2002) Association of depressive syndrome and early deaths among patients after stem-cell transplantation for malignant diseases. *J. Clin. Oncol.*, **20**, 2118–2126.
22. Yirmiya, R., Weidenfeld, J., Pollak, Y. *et al.* (1999) Cytokines, 'depression due to a general medical condition', and antidepressant drugs. *Adv. Exp. Med. Biol.*, **461**, 283–316.
23. McDaniel, J.S., Musselman, D.L., Porter, M.R. *et al.* (1995) Depression in patients with cancer. Diagnosis, biology, and treatment. *Arch. Gen. Psychiatry*, **52**, 89–99.
24. Raison, C.L., Woolwine, B.J., Demetrashvili, M.F. *et al.* (2007) Paroxetine for prevention of depressive symptoms induced by interferon-alpha and ribavirin for hepatitis C. *Aliment. Pharmacol. Ther.*, **25**, 1163–1174.
25. Kent, S., Bluthe, R.M., Kelley, K.W. and Dantzer, R. (1992) Sickness behavior as a new target for drug development. *Trends Pharmacol. Sci.*, **13**, 24–28.
26. Plotkin, S.R., Banks, W.A. and Kastin, A.J. (1996) Comparison of saturable transport and extracellular pathways in the passage of interleukin-1 alpha across the blood-brain barrier. *J. Neuroimmunol.*, **67**, 41–47.
27. Rivest, S., Lacroix, S., Vallieres, L. *et al.* (2000) How the blood talks to the brain parenchyma and the paraventricular nucleus of the hypothalamus during systemic inflammatory and infectious stimuli. *Proc. Soc. Exp. Biol. Med.*, **223**, 22–38.
28. Watkins, L.R., Goehler, L.E., Relton, J.K. *et al.* (1995) Blockade of interleukin-1 induced hyperthermia by subdiaphragmatic vagotomy: evidence for vagal mediation of immune-brain communication. *Neurosci. Lett.*, **183**, 27–31.

29. D'Mello, C., Le, T. and Swain, M.G. (2009) Cerebral microglia recruit monocytes into the brain in response to tumor necrosis factor-alpha signaling during peripheral organ inflammation. *J. Neurosci.*, **29**, 2089–2102.

30. Benveniste, E.N. (1998) Cytokine actions in the central nervous system. *Cytokine Growth Factor Rev.*, **9**, 259–275.

31. Capuron, L. and Dantzer, R. (2003) Cytokines and depression: the need for a new paradigm. *Brain Behav. Immun.*, **17** (Suppl. 1), S119–S124.

32. Kiecolt-Glaser, J.K. and Glaser, R. (2002) Depression and immune function: central pathways to morbidity and mortality. *J. Psychosom. Res.*, **53**, 873–876.

33. Raison, C.L. and Miller, A.H. (2003) Depression in cancer: new developments regarding diagnosis and treatment. *Biol. Psychiatry*, **54**, 283–294.

34. Bower, J.E., Ganz, P.A., Aziz, N. and Fahey, J.L. (2002) Fatigue and proinflammatory cytokine activity in breast cancer survivors. *Psychosom. Med.*, **64**, 604–611.

35. Greenberg, D.B., Gray, J.L., Mannix, C.M. *et al.* (1993) Treatment-related fatigue and serum interleukin-1 levels in patients during external beam irradiation for prostate cancer. *J. Pain Symptom Manage.*, **8**, 196–200.

36. Rigas, J.R., Hoopes, P.J., Meyer, L.A. *et al.* (1998) Fatigue linked to plasma cytokines in patients with lung cancer undergoing combined modality therapy. *Proc. Am. Soc. Clin. Oncol.*, **17**, 68.

37. Butler, L.D., Mohler, K.M., Layman, N.K. *et al.* (1989) Interleukin-2 induced systemic toxicity: induction of mediators and immunopharmacologic intervention. *Immunopharmacol. Immunotoxicol.*, **11**, 445–487.

38. Raab, C., Weidmann, E., Schmidt, A. *et al.* (1999) The effects of interleukin-2 treatment on endothelin and the activation of the hypothalamic-pituitary-adrenal axis. *Clin. Endocrinol.*, **50**, 37–44.

39. Taylor, J.L. and Grossenberg, S.E. (1998) The effects of interferon-alpha on the production and action of other cytokines. *Semin. Oncol.*, **25** (Suppl. 1), 23–29.

40. Lewis, A.M., Varghese, S., Xu, H. and Alexander, H.R. (2006) Interleukin-1 and cancer progression: the emerging role of interleukin-1 receptor antagonist as a novel therapeutic agent in cancer treatment. *J. Transl. Med.*, **4**, 48.

41. Jones, S.A., Horiuchi, S., Topley, N. *et al.* (2001) The soluble interleukin 6 receptor: mechanisms of production and implications in disease. *FASEB J.*, **15**, 43–58.

42. Zins, K., Abraham, D., Sioud, M. and Aharinejad, S. (2007) Colon cancer cell-derived tumor necrosis factor-alpha mediates the tumor growth-promoting response in macrophages by up-regulating the colony-stimulating factor-1 pathway. *Cancer Res.*, **67**, 1038–1045.

43. Aderka, D., Englemann, H., Hornik, V. *et al.* (1991) Increased serum levels of soluble receptors for tumor necrosis factor in cancer patients. *Cancer Res.*, **51**, 5602–5607.

44. Trichopoulos, D., Psaltopoulou, T., Orfanos, P. *et al.* (2006) Plasma C-reactive protein and risk of cancer: a prospective study from Greece. *Cancer Epidemiol. Biomarkers Prev.*, **15**, 381–384.

45. Besedovsky, H., del Rey, A., Sorkin, E. and Dinarello, C.A. (1986) Immunoregulatory feedback between interleukin-1 and glucocorticoid hormones. *Science*, **233**, 652–654.

46. Rivier, C. (1995) Influence of immune signals on the hypothalamic-pituitary axis of the rodent. *Front. Neuroendocrinol.*, **16**, 151–182.

47. Owens, M.J. and Nemeroff, C.B. (1991) Physiology and pharmacology of corticotropin-releasing factor. *Pharmacol. Rev.*, **43**, 425–473.

48. Holsboer, F. and Barden, N. (1996) Antidepressants and hypothalamic-pituitary-adrenocortical regulation. *Endocr. Rev.*, **17**, 187–205.

49. Owens, M.J. and Nemeroff, C.B. (1993) The role of corticotropin-releasing factor in the pathophysiology of affective and anxiety disorders: laboratory and clinical studies. *Ciba Found. Symp.*, **172**, 296–308.

50. Swanson, L.W., Sawchenko, P.E., Rivier, J. and Vale, W. (1983) Organization of ovine corticotropin-releasing factor immunoreactive cells and fibers in the rat brain: an immunohistochemical study. *Neuroendocrinology*, **36**, 165–186.

51. Vale, W., Spiess, J., Rivier, C. and Rivier, J. (1981) Characterization of a 41 residue ovine hypothalamic peptide that stimulates secretion of corticotropin of beta-endorphin. *Science*, **213**, 1394–1397.

52. Musselman, D., Lawson, D. and Miller, A. (2002) Current management of depression in cancer patients: the Schwartz/Lander/Chochinov article reviewed. *Oncology*, **16**, 1110–1115.

53. Capuron, L., Raison, C.L., Musselman, D.L. *et al.* (2003) Association of exaggerated HPA axis response to the initial injection of interferon-alpha with development of depression during interferon-alpha therapy. *Am. J. Psychiatry*, **160**, 1342–1345.

54. Capuron, L., Neurauter, G., Musselman, D.L. *et al.* (2003) Interferon-alpha-induced changes in tryptophan metabolism: relationship to depression and paroxetine treatment. *Biol. Psychiatry*, **54**, 906–914.

55. Capuron, L., Ravaud, A., Neveu, P.J. *et al.* (2002) Association between decreased serum tryptophan concentrations and depressive symptoms in cancer patients undergoing cytokine therapy. *Mol. Psychiatry*, **7**, 468–473.
56. Dunn, A.J., Wang, J. and Ando, T. (1999) Effects of cytokines on cerebral neurotransmission: Comparison with the effects of stress. *Adv. Exp. Med. Biol.*, **461**, 117–127.
57. Lestage, J., Verrier, D., Palin, K. and Dantzer, R. (2002) The enzyme indoleamine 2,3-dioxygenase is induced in the mouse brain in response to peripheral administration of lipopolysaccharide and superantigen. *Brain. Behav. Immun.*, **16**, 596–601.
58. Liebau, C., Merk, H., Schmidt, S. *et al.* (2002) Interleukin-12 and interleukin-18 change ICAM-I expression, and enhance natural killer cell mediated cytolysis of human osteosarcoma cells. *Cytokines Cell. Mol. Ther.*, **7**, 135–142.
59. Moore, P., Landolt, H.P., Seifritz, E. *et al.* (2000) Clinical and physiological consequences of rapid tryptophan depletion. *Neuropsychopharmacology*, **23**, 601–622.
60. O'Connor, J.C., Lawson, M.A., Andre, C. *et al.* (2009) Lipopolysaccharide-induced depressive-like behavior is mediated by indoleamine 2,3-dioxygenase activation in mice. *Mol. Psychiatry*, **14**, 511–522.
61. Raison, C.L., Dantzer, R., Kelley, K.W. *et al.* CSF concentrations of brain tryptophan and kynurenines during immune stimulation with IFN-alpha: relationship to CNS immune responses and depression. *Mol. Psychiatry*, **15**, 393–403.
62. Wichers, M.C., Koek, G.H., Robaeys, G. *et al.* (2005) IDO and interferon-alpha-induced depressive symptoms: a shift in hypothesis from tryptophan depletion to neurotoxicity. *Mol. Psychiatry*, **10**, 538–544.
63. Zhu, C.B., Blakely, R.D. and Hewlett, W.A. (2006) The proinflammatory cytokines interleukin-1beta and tumor necrosis factor-alpha activate serotonin transporters. *Neuropsychopharmacology*, **31**, 2121–2131.
64. Zhu, C.B., Carneiro, A.M., Dostmann, W.R. *et al.* (2005) p38 MAPK activation elevates serotonin transport activity via a trafficking-independent, protein phosphatase 2A-dependent process. *J. Biol. Chem.*, **280**, 15649–15658.
65. Willeit, M., Sitte, H.H., Thierry, N. *et al.* (2008) Enhanced serotonin transporter function during depression in seasonal affective disorder. *Neuropsychopharmacology*, **33**, 1503–1513.
66. Sanchez, M.M., Alagbe, O., Felger, J.C. *et al.* (2007) Activated p38 MAPK is associated with decreased CSF 5-HIAA and increased

maternal rejection during infancy in young adult rhesus monkeys. *Mol. Psychiatry*, **12**, 895–897.

67. Maestripieri, D., Higley, J.D., Lindell, S.G. *et al.* (2006) Early maternal rejection affects the development of monoaminergic systems and adult abusive parenting in rhesus macaques (Macaca mulatta). *Behav. Neurosci.*, **120**, 1017–1024.

68. Miller, A.H. (2009) Mechanisms of cytokine-induced behavioral changes: psychoneuroimmunology at the translational interface. *Brain Behav. Immun.*, **23**, 149–158.

69. Capuron, L. and Miller, A.H. (2004) Cytokines and psychopathology: lessons from interferon-alpha. *Biol. Psychiatry*, **56**, 819–824.

70. Horikawa, N., Yamazaki, T., Sagawa, M. and Nagata, T. (1999) A case of akathisia during interferon-alpha therapy for chronic hepatitis type C. *Gen. Hosp. Psychiatry*, **21**, 134–135.

71. Kamata, M., Higuchi, H., Yoshimoto, M. *et al.* (2000) Effect of single intracerebroventricular injection of alpha-interferon on monoamine concentrations in the rat brain. *Eur. Neuropsychopharmacol.*, **10**, 129–132.

72. Kumai, T., Tateishi, T., Tanaka, M. *et al.* (2000) Effect of interferon-alpha on tyrosine hydroxylase and catecholamine levels in the brain of rats. *Life Sci.*, **67**, 663–669.

73. Schaefer, M., Schwaiger, M., Pich, M. *et al.* (2003) Neurotransmitter changes by interferon-alpha and therapeutic implications. *Pharmacopsychiatry*, **36** (Suppl. 3), S203–S206.

74. Shuto, H., Kataoka, Y., Horikawa, T. *et al.* (1997) Repeated interferon-alpha administration inhibits dopaminergic neural activity in the mouse brain. *Brain Res.*, **747**, 348–351.

75. Sunami, M., Nishikawa, T., Yorogi, A. and Shimoda, M. (2000) Intravenous administration of levodopa ameliorated a refractory akathisia case induced by interferon-alpha. *Clin. Neuropharmacol.*, **23**, 59–61.

76. Grace, A.A. (2002) Dopamine, in *Neuropsychopharmacology: The Fifth Generation of Progress* (eds. K.L. Davis, D.S. Charney, J.T. Coyle and C.B. Nemeroff), Lippincott Williams and Wilkins, Philadelphia, pp. 119–132.

77. Roth, R.H. and Elsworth, J.D. (1995) Biochemical pharmacology of midbrain dopamine neurons, in *Psychopharmacology: The Fourth Generation of Progress* (eds. F.E. Bloom and D.J. Kupfer), Lippincott Williams and Wilkins, Philadelphia.

78. Rye, D.B. (2004) The two faces of Eve: dopamine's modulation of wakefulness and sleep. *Neurology, 63*, **8** (Suppl. 3), S2–S7.

79. Salamone, J.D., Correa, M., Mingote, S.M. and Weber, S.M. (2005) Beyond the reward hypothesis: alternative functions of nucleus accumbens dopamine. *Curr. Opin. Pharmacol.*, **5**, 34–41.

80. Schultz, W. (2007) Multiple dopamine functions at different time courses. *Annu. Rev. Neurosci.*, **30**, 259–288.

81. Capuron, L., Pagnoni, G., Demetrashvili, M.F. *et al.* (2007) Basal ganglia hypermetabolism and symptoms of fatigue during interferon-alpha therapy. *Neuropsychopharmacology*, **32**, 2384–2392.

82. Lou, J.S., Kearns, G., Benice, T. *et al.* (2003) Levodopa improves physical fatigue in Parkinson's disease: a double-blind, placebo-controlled, crossover study. *Mov. Disord.*, **18**, 1108–1114.

83. Wu, H.Q., Rassoulpour, A. and Schwarcz, R. (2007) Kynurenic acid leads, dopamine follows: a new case of volume transmission in the brain? *J. Neural Transm.*, **114**, 33–41.

84. Papanicolaou, D.A. (2000) Euthyroid sick syndrome and the role of cytokines. *Rev. Endocrinol Metab. Dis.*, **1**, 43–48.

85. Raber, J., Koob, G.F. and Bloom, F.E. (1995) Interleukin-2 (IL-2) induces corticotropin-releasing factor (CRF) release from the amygdala and involves a nitric oxide-mediated signaling: comparison with the hypothalamic response. *J. Pharmacol. Exper. Ther.*, **272**, 815–824.

86. Lacosta, S., Merali, Z. and Anisman, H. (2000) Central monoamine activity following acute and repeated systemic interleukin-2 administration. *Neuroimmunomodulation*, **8**, 83–90.

87. Witzke, O., Winterhagen, T., Saller, B. *et al.* (2001) Transient stimulatory effects on pituitary-thyroid axis in patients treated with interleukin-2. *Thyroid*, **11**, 665–670.

88. Musselman, D.L. and Nemeroff, C.B. (1996) Depression and endocrine disorders: focus on the thyroid and adrenal system. *Br. J. Psychiatry,* **168** (Suppl. 30), 123–128.

89. Capuron, L., Gumnick, J.F., Musselman, D.L. *et al.* (2002) Neurobehavioral effects of interferon-alpha in cancer patients: phenomenology and paroxetine responsiveness of symptom dimensions. *Neuropsychopharmacology*, **26**, 643–652.

90. Cleeland, C.S., Bennett, G.J., Dantzer, R. *et al.* (2003) Are the symptoms of cancer and cancer treatment due to a shared biologic mechanism? A cytokine-immunologic model of cancer symptoms. *Cancer*, **97**, 2919–2925.

91. Schubert, C., Hong, S., Natarajan, L. *et al.* (2007) The association between fatigue and inflammatory marker levels in cancer patients: a quantitative review. *Brain Behav. Immun.*, **21**, 413–427.

92. Morrow, G.R., Hickok, J.T., Roscoe, J.A. *et al.* (2003) Differential effects of paroxetine on fatigue and depression: a randomized, double-blind trial from the University of Rochester Cancer Center Community Clinical Oncology Program. *J. Clin. Oncol.*, **21**, 4635–4641.

93. Royster, E.B., Graciaa, D.S., Trimble, L.M. *et al.* (2009) Activation of neuroendocrine pathways by IL-2 administration in patients with malignant melanoma. *Annual Scientific Convention and Program of the Society of Biological Psychiatry*, 67.

94. Nicolson, S., Miller, A., Lawson, D. and Musselman, D. (2006) Neuropsychiatric effects of IL-2: mechanisms and treatment implications. *Depression: Mind Body*, **2**, 120–129.

95. Miller, A.H., Ancoli-Israel, S., Bower, J.E. *et al.* (2008) Neuroendocrine-immune mechanisms of behavioral comorbidities in patients with cancer. *J. Clin. Oncol.*, **26**, 971–982.

96. Andersen, B.L., Farrar, W.B., Golden-Kreutz, D. *et al.* (2007) Distress reduction from a psychological intervention contributes to improved health for cancer patients. *Brain Behav. Immun.*, **21**, 953–961.

97. Gielissen, M.F., Verhagen, S., Witjes, F. and Bleijenberg, G. (2006) Effects of cognitive behavior therapy in severely fatigued disease-free cancer patients compared with patients waiting for cognitive behavior therapy: a randomized controlled trial. *J. Clin. Oncol.*, **24**, 4882–4887.

98. Andersen, B.L., Farrar, W.B., Golden-Kreutz, D.M. *et al.* (2004) Psychological, behavioral, and immune changes after a psychological intervention: a clinical trial. *J. Clin. Oncol.*, **22**, 3570–3580.

99. Antoni, M.H., Wimberly, S.R., Lechner, S.C. *et al.* (2006) Reduction of cancer-specific thought intrusions and anxiety symptoms with a stress management intervention among women undergoing treatment for breast cancer. *Am. J. Psychiatry*, **163**, 1791–1797.

100. Carlson, L.E., Speca, M., Patel, K.D. and Goodey, E. (2003) Mindfulness-based stress reduction in relation to quality of life, mood, symptoms of stress, and immune parameters in breast and prostate cancer outpatients. *Psychosom. Med.*, **65**, 571–581.

101. Courneya, K.S., Mackey, J.R., Bell, G.J. *et al.* (2003) Randomized controlled trial of exercise training in postmenopausal breast cancer survivors: cardiopulmonary and quality of life outcomes. *J. Clin. Oncol.*, **21**, 1660–1668.

102. Cruess, D.G., Antoni, M.H., McGregor, B.A. *et al.* (2000) Cognitive-behavioral stress management reduces serum cortisol by enhancing benefit finding among women being treated for early stage breast cancer. *Psychosom. Med.*, **62**, 304–308.

103. Fairey, A.S., Courneya, K.S., Field, C.J. *et al.* (2005) Effect of exercise training on C-reactive protein in postmenopausal breast cancer survivors: a randomized controlled trial. *Brain Behav. Immun.*, **19**, 381–388.

104. Frank, E. (2007) Interpersonal and social rhythm therapy: a means of improving depression and preventing relapse in bipolar disorder. *J. Clin. Psychol.*, **63**, 463–473.

105. Jacobsen, P.B., Meade, C.D., Stein, K.D. *et al.* (2002) Efficacy and costs of two forms of stress management training for cancer patients undergoing chemotherapy. *J. Clin. Oncol.*, **20**, 2851–2862.

106. McGregor, B.A., Antoni, M.H., Boyers, A. *et al.* (2004) Cognitive-behavioral stress management increases benefit finding and immune function among women with early-stage breast cancer. *J. Psychosom. Res.*, **56**, 1–8.

107. Pinto, B.M., Frierson, G.M., Rabin, C. *et al.* (2005) Home-based physical activity intervention for breast cancer patients. *J. Clin. Oncol.*, **23**, 3577–3587.

108. Stanton, A.L., Ganz, P.A., Kwan, L. *et al.* (2005) Outcomes from the Moving Beyond Cancer psychoeducational, randomized, controlled trial with breast cancer patients. *J. Clin. Oncol.*, **23**, 6009–6018.

109. Irwin, M.R., Cole, J.C. and Nicassio, P.M. (2006) Comparative meta-analysis of behavioral interventions for insomnia and their efficacy in middle-aged adults and in older adults 55 + years of age. *Health Psychol.*, **25**, 3–14.

110. Savard, J. and Morin, C.M. (2001) Insomnia in the context of cancer: a review of a neglected problem. *J. Clin. Oncol.*, **19**, 895–908.

111. Savard, J., Simard, S., Ivers, H. and Morin, C.M. (2005) Randomized study on the efficacy of cognitive-behavioral therapy for insomnia secondary to breast cancer, part II: Immunologic effects. *J. Clin. Oncol.*, **23**, 6097–6106.

112. Davidson, J.R., Waisberg, J.L., Brundage, M.D. and MacLean, A.W. (2001) Nonpharmacologic group treatment of insomnia: a preliminary study with cancer survivors. *Psycho-oncology*, **10**, 389–397.

113. Quesnel, C., Savard, J., Simard, S. *et al.* (2003) Efficacy of cognitive-behavioral therapy for insomnia in women treated for nonmetastatic breast cancer. *J. Consult. Clin. Psychol.*, **71**, 189–200.

114. Zobel, A.W., Nickel, T., Kunzel, H.E. *et al.* (2000) Effects of the high-affinity corticotropin-releasing hormone receptor 1 antagonist R121919 in major depression: the first 20 patients treated. *J. Psychiatr. Res.*, **34**, 171–181.

115. Miller, A.H., Vogt, G.J. and Pearce, B.D. (2002) The phosphodiesterase type 4 inhibitor, rolipram, enhances glucocorticoid receptor function. *Neuropsychopharmacology*, **27**, 939–948.

116. Auyeung, S.F., Long, Q., Royster, E.B. *et al.* (2009) Sequential multiple-assignment randomized trial design of neurobehavioral treatment for patients with metastatic malignant melanoma undergoing high-dose interferon-alpha therapy. *Clin. Trials*, **6**, 480–490.

117. Meyers, C.A., Weitzner, M.A., Valentine, A.D. and Levin, V.A. (1998) Methylphenidate therapy improves cognition, mood, and function of brain tumor patients. *J. Clin. Oncol.*, **16**, 2522–2527.

118. Weitzner, M.A., Meyers, C.A. and Valentine, A.D. (1995) Methylphenidate in the treatment of neurobehavioral slowing associated with cancer and cancer treatment. *J. Neuropsychiatry Clin. Neurosci.*, **7**, 347–350.

119. Dhillon, A.S., Hagan, S., Rath, O. and Kolch, W. (2007) MAP kinase signalling pathways in cancer. *Oncogene*, **26**, 3279–3290.

120. Surh, Y.J. (2003) Cancer chemoprevention with dietary phytochemicals. *Nat. Rev. Cancer*, **3**, 768–780.

121. Monk, J.P., Phillips, G., Waite, R. *et al.* (2006) Assessment of tumor necrosis factor alpha blockade as an intervention to improve tolerability of dose-intensive chemotherapy in cancer patients. *J. Clin. Oncol.*, **24**, 1852–1859.

122. Canaple, L., Kakizawa, T. and Laudet, V. (2003) The days and nights of cancer cells. *Cancer Res.*, **63**, 7545–7552.

123. Liu, L., Marler, M.R., Parker, B.A. *et al.* (2005) The relationship between fatigue and light exposure during chemotherapy. *Support. Care Cancer*, **13**, 1010–1017.

CHAPTER 4

Recognition of Depression and Methods of Depression Screening in People with Cancer

Steven D. Passik and Amy E. Lowery

Department of Psychiatry and Behavioral Sciences,
Memorial Sloan-Kettering Cancer Center, New York, NY, USA

Recent estimates indicate that there are over 10 million cancer survivors in the United States [1]. With cancer becoming a more chronic and survivable disease, quality of life and psychological issues have become even more central and important.

Patients with cancer often experience elevated levels of emotional distress as they adjust to the diagnosis, the side effects of treatments (such as chemotherapy and radiation therapy) and the burden of symptoms caused by the disease itself [2]. Greater attention is now being paid to the emotional needs of cancer patients than in the past. Cancer centers are more focused on the comprehensive needs of these individuals, as healthcare shifts from a biomedical standpoint to a biopsychosocial one [3–5].

Depression is a common problem in cancer patients, which negatively affects their quality of life, physical activities, relationships and

Depression and Cancer Edited by David W. Kissane, Mario Maj and Norman Sartorius
© 2011 John Wiley & Sons, Ltd

sleep. It has been found to reduce compliance with treatment recommendations [6] and can be associated with shorter length of survival [7–10]. Nevertheless, depression is often missed and therefore undertreated [11].

A study examining the ability of physicians to recognize depression in a large sample of ambulatory cancer patients [12] found little concordance between physician estimates of depression and patient ratings. Less than 13% of patients with moderate to severe depressive symptoms were classified as such by physicians, with more than half of these patients being classified as having no significant depressive symptoms.

Depression can be difficult to assess in cancer patients, because depressive symptoms occur on a continuum that ranges from normal feelings of sadness to a major affective disorder. For example, one study examining the differing levels of depression in cancer patients [13] found that 17.9% of the sample scored in the mild range of depressive symptoms, 8.4% scored in the moderate range, and 4.8% scored in the severe range. In total, 31.1% of the sample reported clinically significant depressive symptoms, with 13.2% in the moderate range or greater. Patients who reported having a caretaker endorsed significantly higher depressive symptoms.

IDENTIFYING MAJOR DEPRESSION IN CANCER PATIENTS

Depression can be conceptualized in two ways: as a category or as a dimension. The categorical perspective views depression as a disorder, while the dimensional perspective views depression as increased levels of depressive symptoms without necessarily constituting a disorder [14]. Within the categorical perspective, depression can be defined by the fulfilment of a set of criteria, such as those of the DSM-IV. The DSM-IV criteria for a major depressive episode include the presence of at least five out of nine symptoms (depressed mood, diminished interest/loss of pleasure in activities, weight loss or gain, insomnia or hypersomnia, psychomotor retardation or agitation, fatigue, feelings of worthlessness or inappropriate guilt, reduced ability to concentrate, recurrent thoughts of death or suicide) during the same two-week period, representing a change from previous functioning. At least one of the symptoms must be either depressed mood or loss of interest or pleasure [15].

Diagnosing major depression in cancer patients can be challenging, because the diagnostic criteria in the DSM-IV include several symptoms that overlap with symptoms of cancer or its treatments (appetite loss, weight loss, sleep disturbance, fatigue, loss of energy, difficulty concentrating, psychomotor retardation) [16]. Therefore, using the DSM-IV criteria to assess depression often produces false-positive cases in this population and may result in the administration of unnecessary or ineffective interventions.

Several alternative approaches have been designed to address this diagnostic issue, such as the inclusive, the exclusive, the substitutive, and the increased threshold approaches. In the inclusive approach, all the symptoms of major depression criteria of the DSM-IV are counted, whether or not they might be attributable to cancer [17]. In the exclusive approach, or Cavanaugh criteria, somatic symptoms are deleted from the diagnostic criteria and two new items are proposed (not participating in medical care in spite of ability to do so; not progressing despite improving medical condition and/or functioning at a lower level than the medical condition warrants) [17]. The substitutive approach, or Endicott criteria, substitutes somatic symptoms with non-somatic symptoms (fearfulness or depressed appearance in face or body posture; social withdrawal or decreased talkativeness; brooding, self-pity or pessimism; cannot be cheered up, doesn't smile, no response to good news or funny situations) [17]. Finally, the increased threshold approach applies high symptom-severity thresholds for somatic symptoms [17].

In a study using item response theory (IRT) analysis to determine which items of all combined criteria were the best indicators of depression [17], the authors found that the somatic symptoms of the DSM-IV diagnostic criteria (appetite loss, weight loss, insomnia, fatigue, loss of energy, and diminished ability to concentrate) may not be useful for diagnosing or assessing severity of depression. In addition, feelings of worthlessness and suicidal ideation were not good indicators of the severity of depression. Data analysis suggested that the two Cavanaugh items (not participating in medical care in spite of ability to do so; not progressing despite improving medical condition and/or functioning at a lower level than the medical condition warrants) and one Endicott item (social withdrawal or decreased talkativeness) may be useful in assessing the severity of depression in cancer patients [17]. Two Endicott items (fearfulness or depressed appearance in face or body posture; brooding, self-pity or pessimism) appeared to be good markers of mild depressive disorders, and the remaining Endicott item (cannot be cheered up, doesn't smile, no response to good news or funny situations) appeared to be a good marker for severe major depressive disorder in cancer patients. Overall, this study indicated that the Cavanaugh and Endicott criteria may be better markers for evaluating depression than the DSM-IV diagnostic criteria, suggesting alternative approaches are needed when assessing depression in cancer patients [17].

In a review of the literature on depression in adult cancer patients from 1965 to 1997, Bottomley [18] found that, on average, one in four cancer patients had elevated depressive symptoms. In a meta-analysis of 58 studies from 1980 to 1994 [19], wide variations in symptoms were reported amongst individual studies. Zero to 46% of cancer patients had a depressive disorder, 0.9% to 49% had an anxiety disorder, and 5% to 50% were found to have psychological distress. The authors found that cancer patients did not differ significantly in anxiety and general distress from the normal population. However, cancer patients endorsed significantly more depressive symptoms.

This wide range of prevalence rates of depression in cancer patients reflects differences across studies in characteristics of the samples recruited, patient status (cancer patients undergoing treatment vs. patients seen at follow-up clinics), and methodology (self-report questionnaires vs. psychiatric interview). These differences were illustrated in a cross-sectional study conducted in England [20]. One hundred and seventy-eight cancer patients were given a self-report measure and a psychiatric interview. Results showed that 48% met the criteria for elevated symptoms based on self-report, whereas only 18% met the criteria for an anxiety disorder and 15% for a depressive disorder with a psychiatric interview. The authors concluded that the prevalence was higher using a self-report measure because too few symptoms were present to reach the threshold fixed by the diagnostic criteria, and those present were not disruptive enough to be scored as positive at the psychiatric interview.

ASSESSING DEPRESSION IN SPECIAL ONCOLOGY POPULATIONS

Geriatric Patients

Identifying depression in elderly patients can be a unique challenge. Elderly patients in general are less likely to present with affective symptoms, such as sadness, anhedonia and worthlessness [21]. Research suggests that symptoms such as general malaise or dissatisfaction, diffuse somatic complaints, general aches or stomach aches, hopelessness, late insomnia, variations in mood throughout the day, anxiety, agitation and loss of sexual interest may better differentiate depression in elderly cancer patients [21].

Measures exist that were developed specifically to assess depression in the elderly, such as the Geriatric Depression Scale (GDS, [22]). However, there have been no measures to date specifically defined, normed and validated on elderly cancer patients.

Paediatric and Adolescent Patients

There are few studies on the diagnosis of depression in paediatric cancer patients. As in adult depression, it is important to distinguish normal sadness that is transitory from irritability, insomnia, lack of self-esteem, anorexia and poor social and/or school adjustment, which may signify depression [14].

Paediatric oncologists are often imprecise or inconsistent in their mental health assessment of adolescent cancer patients. A study of 41 cancer patients aged 12 to 19 years found that, while physicians seemed to recognize those who reported clinically significant symptoms of depression and anxiety, they also reported many more of their patients to have psychological distress than patient measures demonstrated [23]. In addition, while physicians accurately recognized overall distress, they did not accurately identify specific symptoms of depression or anxiety. The authors concluded that, while the symptoms patients report may be real, patients may understand them as normative reactions to the unusual life stress of childhood cancer, and may not feel as if they need additional help with management of these feelings [23].

Neuro-Oncology Patients

Patients with brain tumours who are depressed may have a variety of symptoms in addition to neurological deficits. A key consideration to diagnosing depression in this population is to distinguish it from apathy [24]. In depression, patients tend to feel an emotional pain, while in apathy they have a lack of feeling, emotion, interest, or concern.

Palliative Care Patients

A literature review on methods of assessing depression in palliative cancer patients [25] found vast differences in the conceptualization of depression and usage of assessment methods. The authors recommended consistency amongst clinicians and researchers on defining depression, determining the adequate number of relevant symptoms to include in the criteria of depression, and achieving consensus on the use of overlapping somatic symptoms. In addition, they recommended establishing severity thresholds to aid in qualifying the level of depression experienced in this highly-symptomatic palliative population [25].

UNDERDIAGNOSIS OF DEPRESSION IN CANCER PATIENTS

Physicians have not shown to be effective in identifying depression in cancer patients [12], and often referrals are not made until the depression has reached an observable crisis [26].

In a study by Sollner *et al.* [27], oncologists correctly recognized the presence of depressive symptoms in only 11 of 30 severely depressed patients. Correct identification was lower in patients with head and neck or lung cancer and in those with lower socioeconomic status. Oncologists' referral for supportive counselling did not correlate with patient symptoms, but rather with more progressed disease and less denial behaviour.

Passik *et al.* [12] found that depression was inaccurately classified by physicians in nearly 90% of their patients. Physician estimates of patient depression correlated most highly with their ratings of patient anxiety, and were rated higher for patients with a diagnosis of lung cancer and/or stage IV disease. Patients prescribed antidepressant medication were rated as significantly more depressed by physicians [12].

In another study, 100 oncology outpatients were given a structured psychiatric interview. Only 14% of the depressed cases had been identified and treated by the existing health care system [28]. Fallow-field et al. [29] monitored physicians as they rated patients' depression. The misclassification rate was 34.7%. The doctors' predominant tendency was to assess depressed patients as not depressed (595 out of 827 patients with high scores were missed). Physicians were all aware that the psychological status of their patients was being assessed and that their interactions were being videotaped. It is likely that the situation is even worse when doctors are not being monitored.

Oncology nurses are often front line in caring for patients, and receive patient referrals earlier in the course of their illness. This offers the potential for nurses to play a key role in the early identification and management of depression. However, surveys of oncology nurses' rates of detection of depression show significant challenges with assessment and referral. McDonald et al. [30] examined the degree to which nurses recognized levels of depressive symptoms in their patients with cancer. Forty clinic nurses rated the depression levels of 1109 patients. Most of the agreement was on the 'none' or 'mild' end of the continuum. Only 14% of moderately to severely depressed patients were classified accurately by nurses, while 53% of these patients were rated as essentially having no depressive symptoms. Nurses' ratings were correlated most highly with patients' endorsement of more obvious symptoms, such as sadness, tearfulness and irritability, while they were less strongly associated with more subtle symptoms, such as concentration difficulties, anhedonia and somatic symptoms. Men were significantly more likely to be inaccurately classified than were women.

A UK study examining how palliative care clinical nurse specialists assess depression in patients with advanced cancer found that 15% reported they never screened for depression and only 54% screened some of the time [31]. Hospital-based nurse specialists screened less frequently than community nurse specialists, and somatic symptoms (e.g. poor sleep, fatigue, changes in appetite) were used to assess depression more often than non-somatic symptoms (e.g. guilt, suicidal thoughts). Barriers to screening noted by nurses were perceived stigma of a depression diagnosis, side effects of antidepressants, and concern regarding addiction to antidepressant medication. Nearly half of the participants reported that they had received no training in screening for depression, and over two-thirds requested further training [31].

Training of nurse specialists has been the focus of recent research. A pilot study evaluating the effectiveness of a communication workshop for ambulatory oncology nurses found that nurses reported increased confidence in detecting and responding to patient depression and believed they would use these new skills to provide better care [32].

Passik *et al.* [33] examined oncologists' and nurses' ability to recognize depressive symptoms in two cases of cancer patients who were interviewed on videotape. The sample of 32 oncologists and nurses was given a one-hour training on using a brief diagnostic interview for meaningful diagnoses vs. adjustment disorder. Overall, the raters did well on both cases, though somewhat better on the less complex case. In the more complex case, agreement was better on the somatic symptoms. More importantly, follow-up one year later showed that oncologists were still utilizing the training and reported feeling fairly confident in diagnosing depressive disorders [33]. The results of the study indicate that oncologists and oncology nurses can improve their accuracy in diagnosing depression in cancer patients through brief didactic training.

BARRIERS TO THE RECOGNITION OF DEPRESSION IN CANCER PATIENTS

Depression in patients with cancer may be overlooked for several reasons. In general, oncology visits tend to primarily focus on physiological treatment and management of its side effects and secondarily on pain and symptom management. Emotional and psychological symptoms may be overlooked or even discounted as expected consequences of having cancer [30]. Many healthcare professionals working with cancer patients believe that depression is a typical reaction to being diagnosed with such an illness and, therefore, do not identify it as a disorder requiring additional treatment. Some clinicians fear fully exploring psychological symptoms at a vulnerable time for patients [14].

The notion that depression is a normal consequence of a cancer diagnosis has several negative implications. Firstly, it trivializes the degree of suffering associated with depression and its deleterious impact on quality of life. Secondly, it ignores the fact that depressive states exist on a continuum and that clinically significant states are amenable to treatment [34].

Lack of physician awareness of depression may contribute to patients' hesitancy to report emotional complaints. Patients may be reluctant to visit their physician for an emotional complaint for fear that it may distract the physician from curative efforts, or they may fear negative cultural attitudes toward depression [12]. In addition, neither the patient nor the physician may suspect that some somatic symptoms may be the result of an underlying depression, rather than their physical illness. Physicians' lack of awareness may also be due to the heavy caseload of patients being cared for by a typical oncologist.

While diagnosing depression can be difficult in any medical setting, oncology physicians and nurses are faced with the further complication of distinguishing symptoms due to the malignancy or associated medical treatments from symptoms due to depression. Loss of appetite because of chemotherapy, fatigue due to cancer, and lack of sleep because of pain are all examples of the problems that confound the somatic symptoms in diagnosing depression [12]. Also, affective symptoms such as sadness, tearfulness and irritability are influenced by situational factors (such as getting bad news) and may not reflect the presence of depression longitudinally [30].

Even though the symptoms listed above tend to be what oncologists and oncology nurses use to identify depression, an accurate diagnosis of depression in patients with cancer may rely more on cognitive symptoms (worthlessness, hopelessness, guilt, suicidal ideation) and anhedonia than somatic or affective symptoms [34]. In a study on the feasibility of a screening tool [13], items tapping hopelessness, anhedonia and apathy were scored highest by patients who were high endorsers of depressive symptoms overall, suggesting these areas may be key indicators of depression in cancer patients.

Passik *et al.* [35] performed a factor analysis of the Zung Self-Rating Depression Scale [36], a depression scale commonly used with cancer patients. Symptoms of manifest depressed mood were separate from the ideational and anhedonia-related symptoms. Along the somatic dimension, eating-related somatic symptoms (weight and appetite loss) were separate from other important somatic symptoms. The neurovegetative symptoms of depression appeared separable from the cognitive symptoms, with the latter being more reliable for diagnostic purposes. The authors concluded that cognitive symptoms may be more relevant to diagnosing depression in cancer patients, despite the apparent tendency for oncologists to place more importance on the mood and somatic symptoms [35].

REFERRAL OF DEPRESSED PATIENTS WITH CANCER

To date, there is little information regarding the proportion of patients being treated for cancer that are referred to or access mental health services. An Australian study assessed the degree to which patients used available supportive services and their level of satisfaction with them [37]. Although over 30% of the patients reported elevated depressive or anxiety symptoms, 75% had not received any supportive services at any time, and very few (6.5%) reported currently using services. Of the patients provided with psychological treatment, most were receiving it from general practitioners (29%), and the majority of patients (86%) found the experience helpful. It was unclear why the majority of patients reporting elevated symptoms did not access mental health support, but the authors speculated that patients not being aware of services available or not seeing them as being beneficial are possible explanations.

In a study by Passik *et al.* [12], 36% of patients were found to have clinically significant depressive symptoms, yet less than 3% were currently seeing a mental health professional. This highlights the need for further efforts to remove barriers to intervention. A later study by the same group [38] involved designing a fluoxetine-based algorithm to help oncologists choose the most appropriate antidepressant medication and to examine the impact of this intervention on depressive symptoms. Thirty-five patients were identified and treated, and an overall reduction in depressive symptoms was found. These results suggest that a screen and intervene approach can be valuable for teaching oncologists to recognize and treat depressive symptoms in their patients.

One Australian randomized controlled trial of providing coordinated psychosocial interventions based on depression screening in an outpatient clinic showed a significant ability to reduce levels of depression over six months [39].

SCREENING FOR DEPRESSION IN CANCER PATIENTS

To maximize the use of limited treatment resources and provide equal access to mental health services, depressed cancer patients need to be reliably identified. Systematically screening cancer patients for depression is more likely to promote equal access to psychological services, whereas relying only on physician- or patient-initiated referrals might fail to identify and/or overlook a substantial proportion of depressed patients who are in need of supportive treatment [40].

The National Comprehensive Cancer Network Distress Management Panel has developed guidelines for identifying and treating distressing symptoms, such as depression, as a standard of care [41]. This includes screening during the initial visit and periodically throughout treatment. Several cancer centers throughout the US and internationally have implemented programs designed to screen for distress and depression [42] by administering self-report questionnaires to all incoming patients. Based on their scores, patients are treated with interventions ranging from psychoeducation to psychotherapy, family therapy, or pharmacology.

Amongst current screening instruments, a structured interview is considered the gold standard. Unfortunately, the lengthy administration time may not be feasible in high volume clinics. In addition, this utilization of professional staff may not be cost-effective. Therefore, self-report measures have gained popularity as an alternative method of screening for depression in cancer patients. However, a review of currently available measures, as well as discussions with cancer treatment providers, suggest that many of these instruments are not without problems. Patient burden in completing the measures, lengthy administration and scoring time, and multiple scales that confuse busy oncologists are just some of the criticisms of existing measures [43]. Shorter questionnaires are often limited by unclear cut-off scores and have not demonstrated strong psychometric properties.

The practice of screening for depression hinges on the setting of cut-off scores for meaningful follow-up and interventions that are tailored to a particular practice setting. Passik *et al.* [44] examined various cut-off scores for two versions of a depression questionnaire. The shorter version omitted items involving physical symptoms and was found to be equally effective. Questionnaires designed to eliminate neurovegetative symptoms of depression, which can be mimicked by medications and symptoms of cancer, may be a more accurate measure of depression in this particular population.

In a systematic review of screening instruments, measures were categorized as ultrashort (one to four items), short (five to 20 items), and long (21 to 50 items) [40]. Advantages and disadvantages of each type of measure were described. Shorter measures are quick and easy to use in busy clinics and require very few resources to obtain, administer and score. They may have high sensitivity for identifying depressed patients, but often lack specificity, resulting in false positives. Also, patients have reported that the few-item questionnaires often do not accurately describe or capture their mood [40]. Longer measures tend to have stronger psychometric properties and assess a broader spectrum of depressive symptoms. However, they are often more costly and time consuming for staff to administer and score and can result in patient burden, especially for patients receiving palliative care or undergoing strenuous treatment. The authors conclude that choosing an optimal screening tool requires a trade-off between a measure with strong psychometric properties and one with a reasonable length [40].

In the above-mentioned systematic review [40], psychometric properties of existing tools used to screen for emotional distress and depression were evaluated based on the number of validation studies, total number of participants, generalizability across all cancers, the quality of the criterion measure used in the validation, and the reliability, sensitivity and specificity of each instrument. When all ratings were found to be high, a judgement was made that the validation of the screening tool was excellent. From the 106 studies evaluated in this systematic review, Table 4.1 lists the findings for the nine scales used most commonly. The Center for Epidemiological Studies-Depression Scale (CES-D, [46]), the Beck Depression Inventory (BDI, [47]) and the General Health Questionnaire (GHQ-28, [48]) all have excellent characteristics, while the Hospital Anxiety and Depression Scale (HADS, [50]) and the Brief Symptom Inventory-18 (BSI-18, [51]) are judged to be quite good. In addition, the HADS had the most extensively studied validation across disease types and stages, languages and cultures. The Patient Health Questionnaire-9 (PHQ-9, [52]) still lacks sufficient validation in cancer patients. Screening instruments that charge a fee (e.g. BDI-II and BSI-18) are not likely to be widely used compared to those that are free.

Certain populations, such as the elderly, may not be adequately screened by current measures. In a study by Watson *et al.* [9], a healthy geriatric sample (over 70 years old) completed a baseline, face-to-face interview and self-report questionnaires. Two weeks later, a geriatric psychiatrist, blinded to initial results, completed a structured diagnostic interview for major and minor depression. Self-report questionnaires, used at recommended cut points, performed poorly in detecting both major and minor depression. Although one in five participants had significant depression as measured by the diagnostic interview, none of them was seeing a mental health specialist. The authors recommended lowering traditional cut-off scores on existing screening measures in order to adequately screen depression in older adults. They also suggested that some older adults may require novel screening interventions.

More recently, questionnaires are being used on a touch-screen computer, further decreasing workload and expense and improving ease of use. The computer application has been found to be acceptable by patients with cancer in the treatment setting, including older patients [53]. This method can direct and regulate the process of responding to items, not allowing for missing data, and has the potential to offer many additional benefits. Once a patient has completed the questionnaire, the results can be immediately scored and disseminated to the appropriate treatment staff to be used during the patient's visit. This will likely improve communication between

Table 4.1 Evaluation of screening tools for depression (adapted from Vodermaier et al. [40])

Measure	Item no.	N studies	N participants	Generalizability	Reliability	Criterion measure	Validity	Judgement
Distress Thermometer [45]	1	15	4088	Yes	Moderate	Moderate	Moderate	Fair
PHQ-9 [52]	9	2	390	Not yet	High	—	—	Unclear
BSI-18 [51]	18	4	10 749	Yes	High	Moderate	High	Good
CES-D [46]	20	4	1002	Yes	High	High	High	Excellent
EPDS [49]	10	4	470	Palliative care	High	High	Moderate	Good
HADS [50]	14	41	10 203	Yes	High	High	Moderate	Good
ZSDS [36]	20	6	1459	Yes	Low	High	Moderate	Poor
BDI [47]	21	4	398	Yes	High	High	High	Excellent
GHQ-28 [48]	28	2	170	Yes	High	High	High	Excellent

PHQ-9, Patient Health Questionnaire-9; BSI-18, Brief Symptom Inventory-18; CES-D, Center for Epidemiological Studies - Depression Scale; EPDS, Edinburgh Postnatal Depression Scale; HADS, Hospital Anxiety and Depression Scale; ZSDS, Zung Self-Rating Depression Scale; BDI, Beck Depression Inventory; GHQ-28, General Health Questionnaire.

patients and their treatment providers, increase patient satisfaction, reduce cost of administrative staff, and allow for patients to receive more timely interventions. This method of administration can also be helpful for patients with special needs, such as deaf patients, and can be presented in different languages, meeting the needs of a diverse patient population.

In an ongoing study examining the impact of depression screening in lung cancer patients [54], participants were screened for depression in the waiting room prior to their medical visit. Depressed patients (as determined by elevated symptoms on self-report questionnaires) were then randomized to one of four groups where their elevated scores were made available to the patient, physician, both, or neither. Results showed an average of less than two recommendations per patient, and no significant difference between the groups in the number of recommendations made during that visit by physicians to depressed patients. This suggests that, while depression screening is necessary in the care of patients with cancer, it is not sufficient for patients to receive the necessary recommendations and referrals for treatment.

CONCLUSIONS

Depression is a debilitating and frequent condition in cancer patients. There is little doubt that it is poorly recognized, poorly treated and often trivialized ('I'd be depressed if I were in Mr. Xs shoes too'). Such attitudes serve to increase suffering by failing to recognize the full impact of depression on the person with cancer. Screening can be an important part of helping to improve the recognition of depression. But, while necessary, it is surely not sufficient in bringing about real change in and of itself. Like in so many therapeutic areas, screening for problems which medical staff members are unprepared to act upon yields little in the way of focused intervention. Several innovative programs around the world have helped to remedy the problem by, for example, following screening with automatic referral to a depression expert staff member (often an oncology nurse), to improve treatment [55]. There is still a need for algorithmic approaches to be followed by oncologists in smaller and less sophisticated settings, where tools that might facilitate triage and treatment can give staff the ability to arrange appropriate follow-up for cancer patients with depression.

REFERENCES

1. National Cancer Institute (2006) *SEER Cancer Statistics Review 1975–2003*, Cancer Statistics Branch, National Cancer Institute, Bethesda.

2. Thune-Boyle, I.C., Myers, L.B. and Newman, S.P. (2006) The role of illness beliefs, treatment beliefs, and perceived severity of symptoms in explaining distress in cancer patients during chemotherapy treatment. *Behav. Med.*, **32**, 19–29.

3. Hwang, S.S., Chang, V.T., Rue, M. and Kasimis, B. (2003) Multidimensional independent predictors of cancer-related fatigue. *J. Pain Symptom Manag.*, **26**, 604–614.

4. Kunkel, E.J., Bakker, J.R., Myers, R.E. *et al.* (2000) Biopsychosocial aspects of prostate cancer. *Psychosomatics*, **41**, 85–94.

5. Syrjala, K.L. and Chapko, M.E. (1995) Evidence for a biopsychosocial model of cancer treatment-related pain. *Pain*, **61**, 69–79.

6. Kennard, B.D., Stewart, S.M., Olvera, R. *et al.* (2004) Nonadherence in adolescent oncology patients: preliminary data on psychological risk factors and relationships to outcome. *Journal of Clinical Psychology in Medical Settings*, **11**, 31–39.

7. Degner, L.F. and Sloan, J.A. (1995) Symptom distress in newly diagnosed ambulatory cancer patients and as a predictor of survival in lung cancer. *J. Pain Symptom Manag.*, **10**, 423–431.

8. Gilbar, O. (1996) The connection between the psychological condition of breast cancer patients and survival. A follow-up after eight years. *Gen. Hosp. Psychiatry*, **18**, 266–270.

9. Watson, L.C., Lewis, C.L., Kistler, C.E. *et al.* (2004) Can we trust depression screening instruments in healthy 'old-old' adults? *Int. J. Geriatr. Psychiatry*, **19**, 278–285.

10. Palmer, J.L. and Fisch, M.J. (2005) Association between symptom distress and survival in outpatients seen in a palliative care cancer center. *J. Pain Symptom Manag.*, **29**, 565–571.

11. Skarstein, J., Aass, N., Fossa, S.D. *et al.* (2000) Anxiety and depression in cancer patients: relation between the Hospital Anxiety and Depression Scale and the European Organization for Research and Treatment of Cancer Core Quality of Life Questionnaire. *J. Psychosom. Res.*, **49**, 27–34.

12. Passik, S.D., Dugan, W., McDonald, M.V. *et al.* (1998) Oncologists' recognition of depression in their patients with cancer. *J. Clin. Oncol.*, **16**, 1594–1600.

13. Dugan, W., McDonald, M.V., Passik, S.D. *et al.* (1998) Use of the Zung Self-Rating Depression Scale in cancer patients: feasibility as a screening tool. *Psychooncology*, **7**, 483–493.

14. Snyderman, D. and Wynn, D. (2009) Depression in cancer patients. *Prim. Care*, **36**, 703–719.

15. American Psychiatric Association (2000) *Diagnostic and Statistical Manual of Mental Disorders*, 4th edn, text revision, American Psychiatric Association, Washington.

16. Weinberger, M.I., Roth, A.J. and Nelson, C.J. (2009) Untangling the complexities of depression diagnosis in older cancer patients. *Oncologist*, **14**, 60–66.

17. Akechi, T., Ietsugu, T., Sukigara, M. *et al.* (2009) Symptom indicator of severity of depression in cancer patients: a comparison of the DSM-IV criteria with alternative diagnostic criteria. *Gen. Hosp. Psychiatry*, **31**, 225–232.

18. Bottomley, A. (1998) Depression in cancer patients: a literature review. *Eur. J. Cancer Care*, **7**, 181–191.

19. van't Spijker, A., Trijsburg, R.W. and Duivenvoorden, H.J. (1997) Psychological sequelae of cancer diagnosis: a meta-analytical review of 58 studies after 1980. *Psychosom. Med.*, **59**, 280–293.

20. Stark, D., Kiely, M., Smith, A. *et al.* (2002) Anxiety disorders in cancer patients: their nature, associations, and relation to quality of life. *J. Clin. Oncol.*, **20**, 3137–3148.

21. Nelson, C.J., Cho, C., Berk, A.R. *et al.* (2010) Are gold standard depression measures appropriate for use in geriatric cancer patients? A systematic evaluation of self-report depression instruments used with geriatric, cancer, and geriatric cancer samples. *J. Clin. Oncol.*, **28**, 348–356.

22. Yesavage, J.A., Brink, T.L., Rose, T.L. *et al.* (1983) Development and validation of a geriatric depression screening scale: a preliminary report. *J. Psychiatr. Res.*, **17**, 37–49.

23. Kersun, L.S., Rourke, M.T., Mickley, M. and Kazak, A.E. (2009) Screening for depression and anxiety in adolescent cancer patients. *J. Pediatr. Hematol. Oncol.*, **31**, 835–839.

24. Litofsky, N.S. and Resnick, A.G. (2009) The relationships between depression and brain tumors. *J. Neurooncol.*, **94**, 153–161.

25. Wasteson, E., Brenne, E., Higginson, I.J. *et al.* (2009) Depression assessment and classification in palliative cancer patients: a systematic literature review. *Palliative Med.*, **23**, 739–753.

26. Zabora, J. (1998) Screening procedures for psychosocial distress, in *Psycho-Oncology* (ed. J.C. Holland), Oxford University Press, New York, pp. 653–661.

27. Söllner, W., DeVries, A., Steixner, E. *et al.* (2001) How successful are oncologists in identifying patient distress, perceived social support, and need for psychosocial counselling? *Br. J. Cancer*, **84**, 179–185.

28. Berard, R.M., Boermeester, F. and Viljoen, G. (1998) Depressive disorders in an out-patient oncology setting: prevalence, assessment, and management. *Psychooncology*, **7**, 112–120.

29. Fallowfield, L., Ratcliffe, D., Jenkins, V. and Saul, J. (2001) Psychiatric morbidity and its recognition by doctors in patients with cancer. *Br. J. Cancer*, **84**, 1011–1015.

30. McDonald, M.V., Passik, S.D., Dugan, W. *et al.* (1999) Nurses' recognition of depression in their patients with cancer. *Oncol. Nurs. Forum*, **26**, 593–599.

31. Lloyd-Williams, M. and Payne, S. (2002) Nurse specialist assessment and management of palliative care patients who are depressed – a study of perceptions and attitudes. *J. Palliative Care*, **18**, 270–274.

32. Brown, R.F., Bylund, C.L., Kline, N. *et al.* (2009) Identifying and responding to depression in adult cancer patients: evaluating the efficacy of a pilot communication skills training program for oncology nurses. *Cancer Nurs.*, **32**, E1–E7.

33. Passik, S.D., Donaghy, K.B., Theobald, D.E. *et al.* (2000) Oncology staff recognition of depressive symptoms on videotaped interviews of depressed cancer patients: implications for designing a training program. *J. Pain Symptom Manag.*, **19**, 329–338.

34. Passik, S.D. and Breitbart, W.S. (1996) Depression in patients with pancreatic carcinoma. Diagnostic and treatment issues. *Cancer*, **78** (Suppl. 3), 615–626.

35. Passik, S.D., Lundberg, J.C., Rosenfeld, B. *et al.* (2000) Factor analysis of the Zung Self-Rating Depression Scale in a large ambulatory oncology sample. *Psychosomatics*, **41**, 121–127.

36. Zung, W.W. (1965) A self-rating depression scale. *Arch. Gen. Psychiatry*, **12**, 63–70.

37. Pascoe, S., Edelman, S. and Kidman, A. (2000) Prevalence of psychological distress and use of support services by cancer patients at Sydney hospitals. *Aust. N. Z. J. Psychiatry*, **34**, 785–791.

38. Passik, S.D., Kirsh, K.L., Theobald, D. *et al.* (2002) Use of a depression screening tool and a fluoxetine-based algorithm to improve the recognition and treatment of depression in cancer patients. A demonstration project. *J. Pain Symptom Manag.*, **24**, 318–327.

39. McLachlan, S.A., Allenby, A., Matthews, J. *et al.* (2001) Randomized trial of coordinated psychosocial interventions based on patient self-assessments versus standard care to improve the psychosocial functioning of patients with cancer. *J. Clin. Oncol.*, **19**, 4117–4125.

40. Vodermaier, A., Linden, W. and Siu, C. (2009) Screening for emotional distress in cancer patients: a systematic review of assessment instruments. *J. Natl. Cancer Inst.*, **101**, 1464–1488.

41. National Comprehensive Cancer Network (2003) *Distress Management Clinical Practice Guidelines*, vol. 1, National Comprehensive Cancer Network, Washington.

42. Zabora, J.R., Loscalzo, M.J. and Weber, J. (2003) Managing complications in cancer: identifying and responding to the patient's perspective. *Semin. Oncol. Nurs.*, **19** (Suppl. 2), 1–9.

43. Payne, D.K., Hoffman, R.G., Theodoulou, M. *et al.* (1999) Screening for anxiety and depression in women with breast cancer. Psychiatry and medical oncology gear up for managed care. *Psychosomatics*, **40**, 64–69.

44. Passik, S.D., Kirsh, K.L., Donaghy, K.B. *et al.* (2001) An attempt to employ the Zung Self-Rating Depression Scale as a 'lab test' to trigger follow-up in ambulatory oncology clinics: criterion validity and detection. *J. Pain Symptom Manag.*, **21**, 273–281.

45. Roth, A.J., Kornblith, A.B., Batel-Copel, L. *et al.* (1998) Rapid screening for psychologic distress in men with prostate carcinoma: a pilot study. *Cancer*, **82**, 1904–8.

46. Radloff, L.S. (1977) The CES-D scale: a self-report depression scale for research in the general population. *Appl. Psych. Meas.*, **1**, 385–401.

47. Beck, A.T., Ward, C.H., Mendelson, M. *et al.* (1961) An inventory for measuring depression. *Arch. Gen. Psychiatry*, **4**, 561–571.

48. Goldberg, D.P. (1978) *Manual of the General Health Questionnaire*, DJS Spools, Sussex.

49. Cox, J.L., Chapman, G., Murray, D. and Jones, P. (1996) Validation of the Edinburgh Postnatal Depression Scale (EPDS) in non-postnatal women. *J. Affect. Disord.*, **39**, 185–189.

50. Zigmond, A.S. and Snaith, R.P. (1983) The Hospital Anxiety and Depression Scale. *Acta Psychiatr. Scand.*, **67**, 361–370.

51. Derogatis, L.R. (2001) *Brief Symptom Inventory (BSI)-18. Administration, Scoring and Procedures Manual*, NCS Pearson, Minneapolis.

52. Kroenke, K., Spitzer, R.L. and Williams, J.B. (2001) The PHQ-9: validity of a brief depression severity measure. *J. Gen. Inter. Med.*, **16**, 606–613.

53. Allenby, A., Matthews, J., Beresford, J. and McLachlan, S.A. (2002) The application of computer touch-screen technology in screening for psychosocial distress in an ambulatory oncology setting. *Eur. J. Cancer Care*, **11**, 245–253.

54. Passik, S., Rogak, L. and Starr, T. (2008) Maximizing utilization of depression screening in lung cancer patients: a randomized trial. Presented at the 5th Annual Conference of the American Psychosocial Oncology Society, Irvine, March 2008.

55. Strong, V., Waters, R., Hibberd, C. *et al.* (2008) Management of depression for people with cancer (SMaRT oncology 1): a randomized trial. *Lancet*, **372**, 40–48.

CHAPTER 5

Impact of Depression on Treatment Adherence and Survival from Cancer

M. Robin DiMatteo and Kelly B. Haskard-Zolnierek

*Department of Psychology, University of California,
Riverside, CA, USA
Texas State University, San Marcos, TX, USA*

There are cognitive, motivational and social mechanisms by which depression, even that which is not solely cancer-related, can diminish self-initiated health behaviour change and adherence to recommended cancer treatments. This non-adherence can potentially threaten a patient's health and healthcare outcomes, and could ultimately influence survival.

Poor mental health can be a barrier to treatment adherence by undermining the understanding and memory, motivation and attitudes, and social support resources that are all essential to achieving adherence. For treatment adherence levels to remain optimal, physicians and other healthcare professionals should carefully enquire about, and if necessary help the patient receive treatment for, symptoms and behaviours of depression.

THE RELATIONSHIP BETWEEN DEPRESSION AND SURVIVAL IN CANCER

A number of studies provide evidence of a relationship between depression and decreased rates of survival after a cancer diagnosis.

Depression and Cancer   Edited by David W. Kissane, Mario Maj and Norman Sartorius
© 2011 John Wiley & Sons, Ltd

One study of breast cancer patients demonstrated that, at five-year follow-up, women with higher levels of depression had a significantly reduced likelihood of survival [1]. In another study following patients from several months to over 10 years after diagnosis, those with a sense of hopelessness/helplessness were found to have a significantly lower survival rate than those without [2]. In a population-based study of over 10 000 participants, cancer patients with depression had a significantly greater risk of death at eight-year follow-up than did those who were not depressed [3].

Although research to date has not specifically examined adherence to treatment as a mediator of the relationship between depression and cancer survival, non-adherence to treatment is likely to contribute to increased cancer morbidity and mortality [4] *and* non-adherence is higher when patients are depressed [5].

This chapter focuses on examining the relationship of depression to patient adherence in cancer treatment, and on explaining the mechanisms that may account for this relationship.

THE CONCEPT OF ADHERENCE IN CANCER TREATMENT

In the broadest sense, the term *adherence* refers to a patient's behavioural response to his or her health professional's recommendations for health and health care [6]. A patient may follow, or not, a clinician's recommendations to change health behaviour and/or to follow a protocol for disease management activities. Health professionals' recommendations can be for primary prevention, such as a low-cholesterol, low-fat diet, and regular exercise, for secondary prevention, including screening for disease, or for tertiary prevention to cure or manage disease progression (e.g. to slow or minimize damage). Disease management activities may include appointment-keeping for medical visits, self-care activities, and following medication schedules for a particular length of time at a specified dosage and frequency [7].

Failure to adhere to treatment is a common patient response in the context of serious illness such as cancer. Recently, meta-analytic work found that, in more serious diseases including cancer, patients who self-reported poorer health were at significantly greater risk of non-adherence than those who reported their health to be good [8]. This finding was even stronger when patients' health status was assessed with objective measures of disease severity.

With less serious conditions (e.g. arthritis, cataracts), patients in poorer health were more likely to be adherent. However, in more serious diseases (such as cancer, heart failure, HIV), patients who were objectively more severely ill (i.e. had poorer health status as assessed by disease stage in cancer, ejection fraction in heart disease, or viral load in HIV), were *less* likely to be adherent to their regimens than those with better health status [8].

Poor treatment adherence may arise for a variety of reasons, including: a lack of full understanding of the meaning and importance of the regimen, having doubts about the efficacy of treatment, experiencing overwhelming side effects and suffering, and the physical and/or psychological demands of facing a serious illness such as cancer.

OUTCOMES AND CONSEQUENCES OF NON-ADHERENCE

Patients' adherence to clinicians' recommendations for health-promoting behaviours and disease treatment are essential for optimal health outcomes. Meta-analytic evidence shows that adherence is significantly correlated with better healthcare outcomes (with a combined effect size, unweighted mean $r = 0.26$). So, there is a 26% difference in positive health outcomes achieved by those whose adherence is high versus those whose adherence is low [9]. The odds of a good health outcome are 2.88 times higher overall when patients are adherent. Across disease conditions and treatment regimens, however, there exists considerable variability in the relationship between outcomes and both adherence and health behaviours.

There are important consequences of non-adherence, which include poor symptom control, disease recurrence, and/or shortened survival time. Ending treatment early or failing to adhere properly can increase the risk of disease recurrence and metastasis [10]. For instance, patients undergoing breast conservation therapy and radiation have been found to have worse survival when they failed to adhere to their radiation protocols [11]. Other research has found that missing appointments was a key predictor of shorter survival time from breast cancer [12], and research on stage III colon cancer has shown increased risk of mortality when patients fail to complete adjuvant chemotherapy [13].

Some standards of care in cancer suggest a required level of at least 80% adherence [14]. This threshold may be similar to that in HIV care, where patients who are more than 95% adherent to their protease inhibitor medication regimen have significantly better outcomes than those with lower rates of adherence [14]. Adherence below the threshold point might actually be dangerous to the patient, such as with the adjuvant therapy of tamoxifen for breast cancer, where greater patient benefits (decreased risk of recurrence) are proposed to occur only after five years of adherence to medication. Many women discontinue tamoxifen sooner, however, often for psychosocial reasons [15]. In the case of oral or intravenous chemotherapy, side effects that influence quality of life contribute to early cessation of medication-taking, and subsequent failure to derive therapeutic benefit [16].

In addition to directly affecting survival, non-adherence can erode trust in the physician-patient relationship, contributing to frustration for both parties. In addition, there are economic costs of unused prescriptions and unnecessary, unproductive, or wasted medical visits.

The relationship between adherence and outcomes is, of course, not perfect and it is not necessarily linear. Kravitz and Melnicow [17] suggested that the adherence and outcome relationship might be curvilinear. In cancer treatment, as in many conditions, it is possible that increasing diligence over health behaviours may contribute to healthier outcomes only to a point. The advantages of health behaviour may follow the threshold model, in which adherence to treatment such as medication, or self-initiated health behaviour change (e.g. regular exercise), may need to exceed a threshold in order to be effective. Once that threshold is reached, however, there may be marginal benefits and the worry and burden of adhering (e.g. food denial, exceptional vigilance for screening) may add so much stress to the patient's life as to reduce its quality.

Perfect adherence to a suboptimal or erroneous treatment may itself threaten health outcomes [18]. Following 'health recommendations' (e.g. some herbal products or alternative medicine 'cures' such as

Laetrile) from unreliable sources may be dangerous and/or substitute for effective treatments [19]. Some 'alternative' or 'complementary' methods can, of course, be quite effective (e.g. acupuncture for the management of chemotherapy symptoms [20]) while others may be used by patients who have abandoned evidence-based treatments [21].

Finally, adherence has a complex relationship to health because it is difficult to separate the benefits of treatment from the benefits of adhering. There is empirical evidence of a 'main effect' of adherence (even to placebo), such that adherence may be better than non-adherence regardless of what is being adhered to [22, 23]. The potential psychological states that underlie adherence and mediate its effects may be very powerful in their contribution to cancer outcomes.

RATES OF NON-ADHERENCE IN CANCER

Despite the central importance to survival and to healthcare outcomes of many health behaviours and medical treatments, more than 20% of cancer patients have been found to be non-adherent to a variety of treatments (including oral ambulatory chemotherapy, radiation and adjuvant therapy) [24]. Of course, the wide variety of treatment regimens in cancer care results in varying adherence rates. Rates of adherence to tamoxifen treatment for breast cancer have been found to range from 69 to 79% (focusing on adherence and persistence over five years of treatment) [25–27]. Adherence to adjuvant chemotherapy amongst lung cancer patients has been 84% for four of six cycles and 50% for all six cycles [28], but other findings suggest that only about 50% of patients follow through with all recommended cycles of chemotherapy for lung cancer [29]. One study of adjuvant chemotherapy treatment for colon cancer showed 78% adherence [13] and, amongst skin cancer patients, 84% of those who survived melanoma conducted self-examinations at least once a year, but only 59% wore sunscreen [30].

FACTORS AFFECTING ADHERENCE

Patient non-adherence to cancer treatments is multi-faceted. Intentional non-adherence in the context of cancer could reflect the patient's choice not to continue treatment, with its attendant side effects, although it was prescribed in order to prevent recurrence and increase chances for survival. A patient might purposely miss follow-up appointments, or take partial doses of a regimen because he or she feels asymptomatic or does not understand or believe in the purpose of the treatment. Unintentional non-adherence can also occur because of some misunderstanding about the regimen (e.g. timing or dosing), forgetting to follow through because of a chaotic lifestyle, competing responsibilities, or a lack of necessary resources. Of course, the line between intentional and unintentional non-adherence may be a fine one, such as in cases of motivated forgetting or allocation of time and money resources to less important, but more pleasurable, activities than chemotherapy.

The Information-Motivation-Strategy Model© (IMS model©) [31] involves three broad categories of factors that can help to guide our subsequent analysis of the mechanisms by which depression can inhibit health behaviour change and treatment adherence in cancer. The IMS model© states broadly that in order to initiate or adhere to a health behaviour or treatment, patients must: (1) *be informed* (i.e. know what health behaviour or treatment they are expected to perform, and the reasons why); (2) *be motivated* (i.e. want to carry out the behaviour; are motivated by their beliefs, expectations, desires, attitudes and feelings), and (3) *strategize* or plan to carry out the behaviour (i.e. possess the emotional, financial, practical and social resources, including social support, necessary to translate the desired behaviour into action) [31, 32]. Many predictors of adherence have been identified in the empirical research literature and fall into these three broad groups of factors; this simple model provides a framework for understanding adherence to treatment succinctly. The IMS model© identifies the cognitive, motivational and resource-related factors that influence adherence, and can organize our analysis of adherence difficulties faced by cancer patients who are depressed.

HOW DEPRESSION CAN AFFECT ADHERENCE IN CANCER

Depression is very common in cancer. As many as one fourth of cancer patients suffer from major depression [33]; also, anxiety may occur alone or in conjunction with depression [34]. Patients who suffer pain, declining physical status, and the need for ongoing active treatment have a significantly higher risk of depression [35].

The relationship between any patient's depression and non-adherence is strong and significant. In meta-analytic work, compared with non-depressed patients, the odds are three times greater that depressed patients will be non-adherent to their medical treatment recommendations. In the case of cancer, psychological, behavioural and biological pathways can be traced from serious illness stressors through the disease course to non-adherence, suggesting that the effects of depression on adherence can involve interactions amongst physiology, behaviour and emotional experience [36]. Depression can interfere with a patient's ability to adhere to medical regimens including both the desire and the ability to manage behaviour change that is vital when facing chronic conditions such as cancer. Major and minor depression alone can substantially impair quality of life and increase disability [37], and when depression is comorbid with other chronic conditions, quality of life can suffer considerably [38]. Depression can appreciably enhance cancer progression indirectly by jeopardizing adherence to essential cancer treatment regimens [33].

When patients are confronted with the challenges of diagnosis of a serious or life-threatening condition, long-term, health-related habits may be even more difficult than usual to change. Patients' patterns of self-initiated, health-promoting behaviours, such as dietary changes and exercise, may be jeopardized by the stress of complex treatment regimens [8, 39]. Social system factors, environmental factors, and coping patterns may combine with new or existing depression to prevent the adoption of health promotion and disease prevention activities and threaten adherence to treatment. Adherence behaviours can become increasingly difficult with deteriorating health [40]. Patients may find themselves doubting the efficacy of treatment, and they may find their interactions with providers becoming more strained as they face treatment frustrations or grow more severely ill [41, 42]. Adherence to treatment may even seem futile, and patients may become more depressed, socially withdrawn, and hopeless (or even ambivalent) about surviving [43]. When patients struggle with serious medical conditions, depression can contribute to many factors that are essential to initiating and

Table 5.1 Ways by which depression affects adherence to anti-cancer treatments

---

Inability to integrate cancer diagnosis and treatment information
Reduced motivation towards self-care; difficulty planning
Negative health beliefs and pessimism about treatment
Avoidance of health-promoting behaviours
Social isolation and withdrawal
Reduced use of community resources
Greater difficulty tolerating treatment side effects
Lack of desire and difficulty cooperating with plans for treatment

---

maintaining health behaviours, as well as processing and acting upon treatment recommendations [44].

The mechanisms by which depression affects adherence, and possibilities for clinical intervention to improve adherence, can be understood within the IMS model$^{©}$ (Table 5.1). Depression can interfere with the three categories of factors – cognitive, motivational and resource-related – that are essential for adherence. As stated, important pathways influencing adherence are: (a) patients' knowledge and understanding about their health, illness conditions, and treatments; (b) patients' self-perceptions and beliefs, desire and motivation to adhere; and (c) the resources and social support that are essential to make adherence and health behaviour possible. Depression that accompanies cancer can diminish patients' willingness and ability to adhere to their treatments and to initiate and maintain lifestyle changes [45]. This impairment can ultimately threaten patients' quality of life, health outcomes, and even survival. Working clinically to address these three elements of care, while also treating patients' depression, is essential to limit the potential compromise of care. Here we offer both empirical clinical research and theoretical argument to support the use of the IMS model$^{©}$ of adherence to care for cancer patients with comorbid depression.

Depression and Cognitive Processes: Effects on Information

A primary determinant of adherence is the patient's knowledge and understanding of the treatment. In cancer care, patients typically must integrate a great deal of information about their disease and treatment interventions, including not only their diagnoses and the reasons for various treatment choices, but also the treatment regimens including medication scheduling, dietary restrictions, and self-care activities, as well as how to cope with side effects and schedules for monitoring and follow-up. Under the best of circumstances, many patients forget what they have been told by their physicians; one study found that patients forgot 50% of what they were told by the time they exited the medical visit [46].

Low socio-economic status and health literacy are serious risk factors for non-adherence. A study of impoverished early stage breast cancer patients being treated with radiation therapy found that only 36% of patients were fully adherent, and predictors of non-adherence that approached traditional significance levels included patients' literacy [11]. When patients are emotionally distressed, the chances of forgetting are significantly increased [47]. A study focused on understanding information-seeking in end-stage cancer found that, when confronted with terminal illness, a patient's motivation to seek information about his/her condition could not be taken for granted and depended upon several factors: patient open-mindedness, medical facts, healthcare professionals' attitudes toward their patients' informational needs, and the hospital social environment [48].

Depression can seriously challenge the *cognitive functioning and information processing* essential for understanding treatments and organizing behaviour. Essential information (such as the reasons for and scheduling of various treatments, and requirements of self-care) may come from many sources, including health professionals, written instructional materials, and the input of family members. Depression and related stress, anxiety and even anger can impair the ability to learn and maintain new behaviours [49] or to undertake complex tasks that require planning and execution [50]. The physical and psychological symptoms that can interfere with mood, such as insomnia, lower energy, functional impairment, and 'vegetative' symptoms, can be confused with or contribute to depression. When patients are distraught over the course of their illness, they may be more likely to forget recommendations, and less likely to ask questions and participate in the medical visit [5, 38, 51]. Lower levels of patient participation are linked to poorer health outcomes [52]. Amongst

advanced cancer patients, for example, depression and anxiety contribute to physical, social, emotional and cognitive functioning
impairments [47]. Even after controlling for the effects of pain and
illness severity, anxiety and depression are independently associated
with cognitive functioning and fatigue amongst cancer patients [53].

Depression and the Motivation to Adhere

Depression is characterized by pessimism about the future and about
the self, which can interfere with health behaviour and adherence
[5, 54]. Commitment to behavioural change requires patient motivation built on beliefs that support adherence. Depression can significantly undermine those beliefs, and can threaten motivation to follow
recommended treatments. The Health Belief Model, for example,
predicts that health behaviour change will occur if a person feels
susceptible to a severe condition, and believes that adhering has more
benefits than costs [55]. Depression can contribute to the belief that
adherence is not worth the trouble associated with it [56]. Depression
can also lead to diminished self-perceptions and limitations in personal self-efficacy, which are essential to behavioural commitment;
patients with more confidence in their abilities to discuss their
treatment with their healthcare providers are more adherent [57].
Moreover, depression can amplify somatic symptoms, causing additional functional disability and further reducing patient motivation to
change behaviour.

Motivation is essential for the achievement of adherence, and
patients' beliefs, attitudes and perceptions are central to their motivation. The discontinuation of tamoxifen is associated with beliefs
that the risks of treatment outweigh the benefits [26, 56]. Patients
who cope with the challenges of illness in a proactive manner, such as
by seeking support and information, actively solving problems, and
expressing concerns, may be more motivated to adhere than those who
avoid the challenges of the illness and treatment [58].

Following cancer diagnosis, patients (typically those who are not
depressed) may be strongly motivated to engage in behaviours
driven by their health beliefs and attitudes about the effects of health
behaviour on disease outcomes. Many initiate stress management,

quit smoking, begin aerobic exercise, and make major dietary changes [59, 60]; for instance, one study showed as many as half of current smokers quit smoking after a cancer diagnosis [61]. The concept of 'teachable moments' has been used to explain how, after experiencing health events such as serious illness, people are motivated to take on health-promoting behaviours [62]. People may engage in exercise, for example, to deal with the physical and emotional effects of cancer. Comorbid depression, however, can carry a substantial illness burden, often generating additional somatic problems such as fatigue, lowered quality of life, impaired social functioning, and disability [63]. Chronic illness can bring about guilt, worry, anger, sadness, confusion and fear [64]. Amongst cancer sufferers and survivors, anxiety, mood disturbance, fear of recurrence, hopelessness, concern for the effects on loved ones, and altered self-image are common, especially amongst those who are depressed [10, 65, 66].

Optimism and positive coping, in short supply when people are depressed, have been explored extensively as mechanisms through which ill individuals can become more emotionally resilient, motivated and better able to cope with cancer. Folkman and Greer [67] identified those who possess a 'fighting spirit', adopting an optimistic attitude and preferring to be well informed and active in decision-making. For cancer patients, optimism predicts improved quality of life, functional status, and the effective management of pain [68]. In general, characteristics such as optimism, hope and positive coping can directly facilitate positive mood and improved physical health through treatment adherence [69]. Development of a 'chaos narrative of illness', involving a story of disorder, distortion and fragmentation, can foster a sense of anguish, threat and feelings of uncontrollability [70]. Depression can contribute to maladaptive physiological effects throughout the disease course, raising both the symptom severity and corresponding treatment complexity, as well as jeopardizing the patient's belief in the efficacy of the regimen.

Depressed individuals who are chronically ill can resort to an avoidant style of coping, limiting their motivation to change. Avoidant coping involves denial, emotional instability, disavowal about the reality of the illness, and other immature defences. As a result, they may fail to adopt necessary healthy behaviours (healthy diet, exercise, adherence to treatment) and incorporate others that are dangerous to health (e.g. smoking, abusing alcohol, abusing psychotropic medications). While problem-focused coping involves taking the steps necessary to influence the disease process, avoidant coping can severely interfere [71]. An approach-oriented style of coping, which involves seeking information and social support, positive reframing, problem solving, and emotional expression, can bolster adjustment to chronic illness [58]. Avoidance is often termed 'harmful coping' because problems are not faced and solutions are not found, contributing to non-adherence [72]. Improving patients' coping strategies, thus, can be effective in reducing symptoms of psychological distress that hinder health behaviour and the management of illness [73].

Depression and Limitations in Strategizing to Achieve Adherence

Living with cancer often involves coping with complex self-management regimens, and with the physical and emotional distress, social isolation, and threats to identity that accompany the illness. These challenges can strongly affect adherence and health behaviour [74]. Treatment of the cancer can be intimidating and require significant effort in managing side effects. Meta-analytic work [8] demonstrates that when patients have cancer, those in worse health are less likely to be adherent than those whose health is better. When patients are severely ill, their efforts at adherence and health behaviour can be easily derailed by the many physical, psychological and practical challenges that accompany illness [39].

Serious illness can interfere with obtaining and taking advantage of necessary resources (e.g. finances, time and access to care). Research in breast cancer, for example, suggests that patients may miss appointments for reasons including work commitments and poor transportation options [12]. Adherence and health behaviour depend significantly upon having the physical and social resources necessary to implement desired health actions. A patient's ability to purchase and prepare healthy food, to allocate time and financial resources to exercise, and to obtain transportation to medical services and treatments are examples of essential resource-related determinants of health. The acquisition and maintenance of resources can be severely threatened by depression, which can interfere with mobilization of energy and resources [75].

Patients who possess less tangible emotional support and have less cohesive families are at greater risk of non-adherence [76]. Greater social support is associated with better adherence to both breast cancer screening [77] and chemotherapy for colon cancer [13]. Depression can lead to significant social isolation, and can threaten social connections that are essential to health, limiting practical support and preventing the use of available resources. The biobehavioural model offers suggestions for potential causal pathways leading from cancer stressors through disease course [10] and argues that the interrelationships between social support and behavioural and biological factors may affect adherence to treatment in acute and chronic medical conditions [78]. Depression can foster withdrawal and a sense of isolation from family and other sources of social support and can prevent an individual from seeking and utilizing resources (such as family assistance with medications and transportation to medical visits). Major depressive disorder, for instance, is associated with decrements in functioning, greater risk of marital distress and missed work, and accompanying threats to resources [79]. Both depression and cancer can foster social rejection and isolation leading to worsening depression and direct threats to adherence [80]. The cumulative experience of illness, depression, family conflict and financial burden may deprive an individual of the capacity to change and adhere to medical recommendations. Amongst older adults with depression, perceptions of stigma can predict medication discontinuation [81].

Finally, it is important that adherence not be unduly difficult for the patient; treatment must fit into the patient's lifestyle if it is to be successful. Adherence is compromised when the regimen is complex or side effects burdensome [57]. In chemotherapy, side effects that harm physical, social and emotional functioning (for example, in breast cancer, hot flushes and joint pain from adjuvant therapy [82]) can contribute to discontinuing the regimen before it has been completed, leading to the failure to achieve optimum benefits [16]. Radiation therapy can be physically and emotionally draining and accompanied by distressing side effects. Chemotherapy can compromise immune functioning, resulting in fatigue as well as the need for social isolation to reduce the risk of infection. The addition of distressing side effects to existing depression can increase the chances of non-adherence.

CLINICAL RECOMMENDATIONS

It is critically important that physicians are aware of how depression in patients with cancer can affect their adherence. Patients should be screened for mental health problems, so that these challenges can be addressed in tandem with guidelines and recommendations for treatment adherence and health behaviour change. A number of specific recommendations for clinical practitioners follow.

First, patients should be helped to adhere by being assisted with the three major components of adherence: information, motivation and strategy. Adherence itself (even to placebo) can have positive effects on health and may provide some clues to the role of psychological states and the effects of cognitive, motivational and resource factors (including social support) to achieve treatment goals. The stress of diagnosis and treatment can affect the most basic aspects of patients' lives, including what they eat, how well they sleep, the degree to which they want to exercise, and their use of substances such as alcohol and tobacco. Adherence to clinicians' recommendations and patients' own self-directed health behaviours may be mutually reinforcing such that adherent patients may take on additional positive health behaviour changes. Their resulting positive expectations may increase their likelihood of further engagement in the care plan [83]. Non-adherent patients, on the other hand, may become defensive as they are further distanced from health information and their physicians, and they may move further away from health-promoting lifestyles [10]. More favourable outcomes can occur because adherent patients benefit from the direct therapeutic effects of their treatments, or possibly also because of the 'non-specific' effects of adhering [23, 84]. Benefits may accrue through biological, pharmacological, psychological and behavioural mechanisms, including optimistic expectations [22].

Second, non-adherence should be viewed as a potential clinical marker for depression. Physicians need to be aware of the strong relationship between non-adherence and depression, and when they recognize that patients are non-adherent, they should screen for depression. Depressed patients should be referred for further mental health interventions. Physicians should follow-up to be sure that these patients receive appropriate treatment for their depression and should assess whether their adherence improves as a result.

Third, providers should foster a strong clinician-patient relationship, effective communication, and partnership. Building the therapeutic relationship will help providers to diagnose and effectively manage both depression and adherence. One of the most important steps to achieving adherence involves the development of rapport through the sharing of goals and hoped-for outcomes. When a patient is motivated to adhere to treatment recommendations, it is ideally (but by no means usually) the case that these choices are mutually decided upon by patients and their physicians through shared decision-making [85]. Demonstrating empathy for patients involves the provider's awareness of the perspective of the patient, understanding the patient's point of view, and communicating that perception to the patient. Such empathic behaviour should extend toward understanding the difficulties of disease management and medication-taking, and should view solving the challenges of adherence from the patient's perspective. By focusing on the patient's experience of and psychological response to illness, patient-centred care helps avoid fragmented care.

Communication is also essential to supporting patients emotionally and helping them find meaning in the illness, helping to balance its negative consequences and improving their adjustment [67]. Individuals who find meaning in their experience may feel a greater sense of control, improved psychological adjustment, better coping, mood and health status [69, 86]. Although research on finding meaning and adherence has not been done on cancer patients, research on patients with tuberculosis and HIV has indicated a significant relationship between assessment of meaning or benefit in life and adherence to treatment [87, 88].

Physicians can also communicate support for patients' positive expectations. The avoidance of pessimism and nurturance of hope promote better health behaviours and greater patient adherence to treatment through increased motivation. Research by Epstein [84] and others [23] suggests that the benefits of adherence occur regardless of whether treatment is an active medication or placebo; in experimental studies, adherence to placebo resulted in lower mortality risk [89]. With new health habits comes greater confidence and a 'self-fulfilling prophecy' may ensue, in which patients' expectations alone drive beneficial outcomes. Self-efficacy expectancies of personal competence, optimism and a sense of well-being may lead to more adaptive physiological and immunological responses. In patients with cardiovascular disease, for example, these self-efficacy expectancies have been shown to play a vital role in persuading patients that they are capable of making healthier dietary choices [90].

Finally, whenever we examine health behaviour change and treatment adherence, we recognize that causal inferences are problematic because patient adherence and health behaviour can be both the cause, and the consequence, of psychological states. Patients might behave in healthy ways because they feel positive and hopeful, or they may feel positive and hopeful because they are behaving in healthy ways; those who are less distressed emotionally may be more likely to adhere, but it is possible that adherence, emotional experience, and health are all caused by another factor entirely (for example, the availability of specific social and financial resources; or individual characteristics such as expectations, locus of control, hardiness and optimism). It is not possible to do a controlled experiment, treating one group to emotional distress and determining its effect. In all research such as this, where randomized experiments and clinical trials are not possible, careful examination of potential conceptual, measurement and methodology artifacts is essential. Meta-analysis can provide one way of systematically examining research on these complex relationships, while also taking into account various methodological, measurement and substantive moderators [91].

It is possible to design interventions that relieve psychological distress amongst patients with cancer, and determine the resultant effects on adherence. In one study of patients with breast cancer, for example, treatment with selective serotonin reuptake inhibitors (SSRIs) resulted in improvements in depression, reduced perceptions of illness severity, and improvement in quality of life [92] (although adherence was not measured as an outcome). Another group therapy intervention for women with advanced breast cancer both ameliorated and prevented depression while promoting adherence to anti-cancer treatments [93, 94]. Interventions to increase patient self-efficacy have been found to significantly improve adherence to pharmacotherapy and resulting depression outcomes [91, 95].

Ideally, further research will identify both mediating and moderating mechanisms in the process of improving health behaviour change and adherence. In the meantime, the IMS model$^{©}$ provides a conceptual framework to guide physicians and other healthcare providers in understanding patient barriers and facilitators to adherence, recognizing the central role played by depression and the need to manage and treat this important comorbid condition.

REFERENCES

1. Watson, M., Haviland, J.S., Greer, S. *et al.* (1999) Influence of psychological response on survival in breast cancer: a population-based cohort study. *Lancet*, **354**, 1331–1336.
2. Watson, M., Homewood, J., Haviland, J. and Bliss, J.M. (2005) Influence of psychological response on breast cancer survival: 10-year follow-up of a population-based cohort. *Eur. J. Cancer*, **41**, 1710–1714.
3. Onitilo, A.A., Nietert, P.J. and Egede, L.E. (2006) Effect of depression on all-cause mortality in adults with cancer and differential effects by cancer site. *Gen. Hosp. Psychiatry*, **28**, 396–402.
4. Kissane, D. (2009) Beyond the psychotherapy and survival debate: the challenge of social disparity, depression and treatment adherence in psychosocial cancer care. *Psychooncology*, **18**, 1–5.
5. DiMatteo, M.R., Lepper, H.S. and Croghan, T.W. (2000) Depression is a risk factor for noncompliance with medical treatment: meta-analysis of the effects of anxiety and depression on patient adherence. *Arch. Intern. Med.*, **160**, 2101–2107.
6. Zolnierek, K.B. and DiMatteo, M.R. (2009) Physician communication and patient adherence to treatment: a meta-analysis. *Med. Care*, **47**, 826–834.
7. Winett, R.A. (1995) A framework for health promotion and disease prevention programs. *Am. Psychol.*, **50**, 341–350.
8. DiMatteo, M.R., Haskard, K.B. and Williams, S.L. (2007) Health beliefs, disease severity, and patient adherence: a meta-analysis. *Med. Care*, **45**, 521–528.
9. DiMatteo, M.R., Giordani, P.J., Lepper, H.S. and Croghan, T.W. (2002) Patient adherence and medical treatment outcomes: a meta-analysis. *Med. Care*, **40**, 794–811.

10. Andersen, B.L., Kiecolt-Glaser, J.K. and Glaser, R. (1994) A biobehavioral model of cancer stress and disease course. *Am. Psychol.*, **49**, 389–404.

11. Li, B.D., Brown, W.A., Ampil, F.L. *et al.* (2000) Patient compliance is critical for equivalent clinical outcomes for breast cancer treated by breast-conservation therapy. *Ann. Surg.*, **231**, 883–889.

12. Howard, D.L., Penchansky, R. and Brown, M.B. (1998) Disaggregating the effects of race on breast cancer survival. *Fam. Med.*, **30**, 228–235.

13. Dobie, S.A., Baldwin, L.M., Dominitz, J.A. *et al.* (2006) Completion of therapy by Medicare patients with stage III colon cancer. *J. Natl. Cancer Inst.*, **98**, 610–619.

14. Paterson, D.L., Swindells, S., Mohr, J. *et al.* (2000) Adherence to protease inhibitor therapy and outcomes in patients with HIV infection. *Ann. Intern. Med.*, **133**, 21–30.

15. Early Breast Cancer Trialists Collaborative Group (1998) Tamoxifen for early breast cancer: an overview of the randomized trials. *Lancet*, **351**, 1451–1467.

16. Richardson, J.L., Marks, G. and Levine, A. (1988) The influence of symptoms of disease and side effects of treatment on compliance with cancer therapy. *J. Clin. Oncol.*, **6**, 1746–1752.

17. Kravitz, R.L. and Melnikow, J. (2004) Medical adherence research: time for a change in direction? *Med. Care*, **42**, 197–199.

18. Kohn, L.T., Corrigan, J. and Donaldson, M.S. (2000) *To Err is Human: Building a Safer Health System*, National Academies Press, Washington.

19. Greenberg, D.M. (1980) The case against laetrile: the fraudulent cancer remedy. *Cancer*, **45**, 799–807.

20. Shen, J., Wenger, N., Glaspy, J. *et al.* (2000) Electroacupuncture for control of myeloablative chemotherapy-induced emesis: a randomized controlled trial. *JAMA*, **284**, 2755–2761.

21. Lerner, I.J. and Kennedy, B.J. (1992) The prevalence of questionable methods of cancer treatment in the United States. *CA Cancer J. Clin.*, **42**, 181–191.

22. Czajkowski, S.M., Chesney, M.A. and Smith, A.W. (1998) Adherence and the placebo effect, in *The Handbook of Health Behavior Change* (eds. S. Shumaker, E.B. Schron, J.K. Ockene and W.L. McBee), Springer, New York, pp. 515–534.

23. Horwitz, R.I. and Horwitz, S.M. (1993) Adherence to treatment and health outcomes. *Arch. Intern. Med.*, **153**, 1863–1868.

24. DiMatteo, M.R. (2004) Variations in patients' adherence to medical recommendations: a quantitative review of 50 years of research. *Med. Care*, **42**, 200–209.

25. Kahn, K.L., Schneider, E.C., Malin, J.L. *et al.* (2007) Patient centered experiences in breast cancer: predicting long-term adherence to tamoxifen use. *Med. Care*, **45**, 431–439.

26. Lash, T.L., Fox, M.P., Westrup, J.L. *et al.* (2006) Adherence to tamoxifen over the five-year course. *Breast Cancer Res. Treat.*, **99**, 215–220.

27. Partridge, A.H., Wang, P.S., Winer, E.P. and Avorn, J. (2003) Nonadherence to adjuvant tamoxifen therapy in women with primary breast cancer. *J. Clin. Oncol.*, **21**, 602–606.

28. Dediu, M., Alexandru, A., Median, D. *et al.* (2006) Compliance with adjuvant chemotherapy in non-small cell lung cancer. The experience of a single institution evaluating a cohort of 356 patients. *J. BUON*, **11**, 425–432.

29. Alam, N., Shepherd, F.A., Winton, T. *et al.* (2005) Compliance with postoperative adjuvant chemotherapy in non-small cell lung cancer. An analysis of national cancer institute of Canada and intergroup trial jbr.10 and a review of the literature. *Lung Cancer*, **47**, 385–394.

30. Manne, S. and Lessin, S. (2006) Prevalence and correlates of sun protection and skin self-examination practices among cutaneous malignant melanoma survivors. *J. Behav. Med.*, **29**, 419–434.

31. Martin, L.R., Haskard-Zolnierek, K.B. and DiMatteo, M.R. (2010) *Health Behavior Change and Treatment Adherence: Evidence-Based Guidelines for Healthcare*, Oxford University Press, New York.

32. DiMatteo, M.R. and DiNicola, D.D. (1982) *Achieving Patient Compliance: The Psychology of the Medical Practitioner's Role*, Pergamon, Elsmford.

33. Spiegel, D. and Giese-Davis, J. (2003) Depression and cancer: mechanisms and disease progression. *Biol. Psychiatry*, **54**, 269–282.

34. Mineka, S., Watson, D. and Clark, L.A. (1998) Comorbidity of anxiety and unipolar mood disorders. *Annu. Rev. Psychol.*, **49**, 377–412.

35. Newport, D.J. and Nemeroff, C.B. (1998) Assessment and treatment of depression in the cancer patient. *J. Psychosom. Res.*, **45**, 215–237.

36. Andersen, B.L., Anderson, B. and deProsse, C. (1989) Controlled prospective longitudinal study of women with cancer: Ii. Psychological outcomes. *J. Consult. Clin. Psychol.*, **57**, 692–697.

37. Wagner, H.R., Burns, B.J., Broadhead, W.E. *et al.* (2000) Minor depression in family practice: functional morbidity, co-morbidity, service utilization and outcomes. *Psychol. Med.*, **30**, 1377–1390.

38. Katon, W.J., Unutzer, J. and Simon, G. (2004) Treatment of depression in primary care: where we are, where we can go. *Med. Care*, **42**, 1153–1157.

39. Brown, C., Dunbar-Jacob, J., Palenchar, D.R. *et al.* (2001) Primary care patients' personal illness models for depression: a preliminary investigation. *Fam. Pract.*, **18**, 314–320.

40. Wagner, G.J. and Ryan, G.W. (2004) Relationship between routinization of daily behaviors and medication adherence in HIV-positive drug users. *AIDS Patient Care STDS*, **18**, 385–393.

41. Hall, J.A., Roter, D.L., Milburn, M.A. and Daltroy, L.H. (1996) Patients' health as a predictor of physician and patient behavior in medical visits. A synthesis of four studies. *Med. Care*, **34**, 1205–1218.

42. Horne, R. and Weinman, J. (1999) Patients' beliefs about prescribed medicines and their role in adherence to treatment in chronic physical illness. *J. Psychosom. Res.*, **47**, 555–567.

43. Christensen, A.J., Benotsch, E.G. and Smith, T.W. (1997) Determinants of regimen adherence in renal dialysis, in *Handbook of Health Behavior Research II: Provider Determinants* (ed. D.S. Gochman), Plenum, New York, pp. 231–242.

44. De Vito Dabbs, A., Dew, M.A., Stilley, C.S. *et al.* (2003) Psychosocial vulnerability, physical symptoms and physical impairment after lung and heart-lung transplantation. *J. Heart Lung Transplant*, **22**, 1268–1275.

45. Katon, W.J. (2003) Clinical and health services relationships between major depression, depressive symptoms, and general medical illness. *Biol. Psychiatry*, **54**, 216–226.

46. Ley, P. and Spelman, M.S. (1965) Communications in an out-patient setting. *Br. J. Soc. Clin. Psychol.*, **4**, 114–116.

47. Mystakidou, K., Tsilika, E., Parpa, E. *et al.* (2005) Assessment of anxiety and depression in advanced cancer patients and their relationship with quality of life. *Qual. Life Res.*, **14**, 1825–1833.

48. Zanchetta, M.S. and Moura, S.L. (2006) Self-determination and information seeking in end-stage cancer. *Clin. J. Oncol. Nurs.*, **10**, 803–807.

49. Spiegel, D. (1997) Psychosocial aspects of breast cancer treatment. *Semin. Oncol.*, **24**, S1–36-S31-47.

50. Wells, K.B. and Burnam, M.A. (1991) Caring for depression in America: lessons learned from early findings of the Medical Outcomes Study. *Psychiatr. Med.*, **9**, 503–519.

51. Sherbourne, C., Schoenbaum, M., Wells, K.B. and Croghan, T.W. (2004) Characteristics, treatment patterns, and outcomes of persistent depression despite treatment in primary care. *Gen. Hosp. Psychiatry*, **26**, 106–114.

52. Chewning, B. and Sleath, B. (1996) Medication decision-making and management: a client-centered model. *Soc. Sci. Med.*, **42**, 389–398.
53. Smith, E.M., Gomm, S.A. and Dickens, C.M. (2003) Assessing the independent contribution to quality of life from anxiety and depression in patients with advanced cancer. *Palliative Med.*, **17**, 509–513.
54. Peterman, A.H. and Cella, D.F. (1998) Adherence issues among cancer patients, in *The Handbook of Health Behavior Change* (eds. S. Shumaker, E.B. Schron, J.K. Ockene and W.L. McBee), Springer, New York, pp. 462–482.
55. Rosenstock, I.M. (1974) Historical origins of the health belief model. *Health Educ. Monogr.*, 2.
56. Fink, A.K., Gurwitz, J., Rakowski, W. *et al.* (2004) Patient beliefs and tamoxifen discontinuance in older women with estrogen receptor-positive breast cancer. *J. Clin. Oncol.*, **22**, 3309–3315.
57. Demissie, S., Silliman, R.A. and Lash, T.L. (2001) Adjuvant tamoxifen: predictors of use, side effects, and discontinuation in older women. *J. Clin. Oncol.*, **19**, 322–328.
58. Holahan, C.J., Moos, R.H., Holahan, C.K. and Brennan, P.L. (1997) Social context, coping strategies, and depressive symptoms: an expanded model with cardiac patients. *J. Pers. Soc. Psychol.*, **72**, 918–928.
59. Blanchard, C.M., Denniston, M.M., Baker, F. *et al.* (2003) Do adults change their lifestyle behaviors after a cancer diagnosis? *Am. J. Health Behav.*, **27**, 246–256.
60. Humpel, N., Magee, C. and Jones, S.C. (2007) The impact of a cancer diagnosis on the health behaviors of cancer survivors and their family and friends. *Support. Care Cancer*, **15**, 621–630.
61. Gritz, E.R., Fingeret, M.C., Vidrine, D.J. *et al.* (2006) Successes and failures of the teachable moment: smoking cessation in cancer patients. *Cancer*, **106**, 17–27.
62. Demark-Wahnefried, W., Aziz, N.M., Rowland, J.H. and Pinto, B.M. (2005) Riding the crest of the teachable moment: promoting long-term health after the diagnosis of cancer. *J. Clin. Oncol.*, **23**, 5814–5830.
63. Spitzer, R.L., Kroenke, K., Linzer, M. *et al.* (1995) Health-related quality of life in primary care patients with mental disorders. Results from the PRIME-MD 1000 study. *JAMA*, **274**, 1511–1517.
64. Bury, M. (1982) Chronic illness as biographical disruption. *Sociol. Health Illn.*, **4**, 167–182.
65. Hatchett, L., Friend, R., Symister, P. and Wadhwa, N. (1997) Interpersonal expectations, social support, and adjustment to chronic illness. *J. Pers. Soc. Psychol.*, **73**, 560–573.

66. Koopman, C., Hermanson, K., Diamond, S. *et al.* (1998) Social support, life stress, pain and emotional adjustment to advanced breast cancer. *Psychooncology*, **7**, 101–111.

67. Folkman, S. and Greer, S. (2000) Promoting psychological well-being in the face of serious illness: when theory, research and practice inform each other. *Psychooncology*, **9**, 11–19.

68. Astin, J.A. and Forys, K. (2004) Psychosocial determinants of health and illness: integrating mind, body, and spirit. *Adv. Mind Body Med.*, **20**, 14–21.

69. Sears, S.R., Stanton, A.L. and Danoff-Burg, S. (2003) The yellow brick road and the emerald city: benefit finding, positive reappraisal coping and posttraumatic growth in women with early-stage breast cancer. *Health Psychol.*, **22**, 487–497.

70. Kleinman, A. (1988) *The Illness Narratives: Suffering, Healing, and the Human Condition*, Basic Books, New York.

71. Schussler, G. (1992) Coping strategies and individual meanings of illness. *Soc. Sci. Med.*, **34**, 427–432.

72. Carver, C.S., Pozo, C., Harris, S.D. *et al.* (1993) How coping mediates the effect of optimism on distress: a study of women with early stage breast cancer. *J. Pers. Soc. Psychol.*, **65**, 375–390.

73. Barton, C., Clarke, D., Sulaiman, N. and Abramson, M. (2003) Coping as a mediator of psychosocial impediments to optimal management and control of asthma. *Respir. Med.*, **97**, 747–761.

74. Jerant, A.F., von Friederichs-Fitzwater, M.M. and Moore, M. (2005) Patients' perceived barriers to active self-management of chronic conditions. *Patient Educ. Couns.*, **57**, 300–307.

75. Reuter, K., Classen, C.C., Roscoe, J.A. *et al.* (2006) Association of coping style, pain, age and depression with fatigue in women with primary breast cancer. *Psychooncology*, **15**, 772–779.

76. DiMatteo, M.R. (2004) Social support and patient adherence to medical treatment: a meta-analysis. *Health Psychol.*, **23**, 207–218.

77. Katapodi, M.C., Facione, N.C., Miaskowski, C. *et al.* (2002) The influence of social support on breast cancer screening in a multicultural community sample. *Oncol. Nurs. Forum*, **29**, 845–852.

78. Gonzalez, J.S., Penedo, F.J., Antoni, M.H. *et al.* (2004) Social support, positive states of mind, and HIV treatment adherence in men and women living with HIV/AIDS. *Health Psychol.*, **23**, 413–418.

79. Olfson, M., Fireman, B., Weissman, M.M. *et al.* (1997) Mental disorders and disability among patients in a primary care group practice. *Am. J. Psychiatry*, **154**, 1734–1740.

80. Fife, B.L. and Wright, E.R. (2000) The dimensionality of stigma: a comparison of its impact on the self of persons with HIV/AIDS and cancer. *J. Health Soc. Behav.*, **41**, 50–67.
81. Sirey, J.A., Bruce, M.L., Alexopoulos, G.S. *et al.* (2001) Perceived stigma as a predictor of treatment discontinuation in young and older outpatients with depression. *Am. J. Psychiatry*, **158**, 479–481.
82. Cella, D. and Fallowfield, L.J. (2007) Recognition and management of treatment-related side effects for breast cancer patients receiving adjuvant endocrine therapy. *Breast Cancer Res. Treat.*, **107**, 167–180.
83. Taylor, S.E., Kemeny, M.E., Reed, G.M. *et al.* (2000) Psychological resources, positive illusions, and health. *Am. Psychol.*, **55**, 99–109.
84. Epstein, L.H. (1984) The direct effects of compliance on health outcome. *Health Psychol.*, **3**, 385–393.
85. DiMatteo, M., Reiter, R. and Gambone, J. (1994) Enhancing medication adherence through communication and informed collaborative choice. *Health Commun.*, **6**, 253–265.
86. Fife, B.L. (1995) The measurement of meaning in illness. *Soc. Sci. Med.*, **40**, 1021–1028.
87. Corless, I.B., Nicholas, P.K., Wantland, D. *et al.* (2006) The impact of meaning in life and life goals on adherence to a tuberculosis medication regimen in South Africa. *Int. J. Tuberc. Lung Dis.*, **10**, 1159–1165.
88. Luszczynska, A., Sarkar, Y. and Knoll, N. (2006) Received social support, self-efficacy, and finding benefits in disease as predictors of physical functioning and adherence to antiretroviral therapy. *Patient Educ. Couns.*, **66**, 37–42.
89. Simpson, S.H., Eurich, D.T., Majumdar, S.R. *et al.* (2006) A meta-analysis of the association between adherence to drug therapy and mortality. *BMJ*, **333**, 15.
90. Newman, S. (2004) Engaging patients in managing their cardiovascular health. *Heart*, **90** (Suppl. 4), iv9–iv13.
91. Rosenthal, R. and DiMatteo, M.R. (2001) Meta-analysis: recent developments in quantitative methods for literature reviews. *Ann. Rev. Psychol.*, **52**, 59–82.
92. Pezzella, G., Moslinger-Gehmayr, R. and Contu, A. (2001) Treatment of depression in patients with breast cancer: a comparison between paroxetine and amitriptyline. *Breast Cancer Res. Treat.*, **70**, 1–10.
93. Kissane, D.W., Grabsch, B., Clarke, D.M. *et al.* (2007) Supportive-expressive group therapy for women with metastatic breast cancer: survival and psychosocial outcome from a randomized controlled trial. *Psychooncology*, **16**, 277–286.

94. Kissane, D.W., Grabsch, B., Clarke, D.M. *et al.* (2004) Supportive-expressive group therapy: the transformation of existential ambivalence into creative living while enhancing adherence to anti-cancer therapies. *Psychooncology*, **13**, 755–768.
95. Ludman, E., Katon, W., Bush, T. *et al.* (2003) Behavioural factors associated with symptom outcomes in a primary care-based depression prevention intervention trial. *Psychol. Med.*, **33**, 1061–1070.

CHAPTER 6

Suicide and Desire for Hastened Death in People with Cancer

William Breitbart, Hayley Pessin and Elissa Kolva

Department of Psychiatry and Behavioral Sciences, Memorial Sloan-Kettering Cancer Center, New York, NY, USA

Cancer patients are more likely to express suicidal ideation and commit suicide than both the general population and other medically ill populations [1–3]. Hence, clinicians working with these patients should be competent in the identification and assessment of those who are at risk for suicide. This chapter presents an overview of the literature on suicide and desire for hastened death (DHD) in cancer [4, 5]. Relevant topics include prevalence, risk factors, assessment of suicidal ideation, as well as clinical guidelines to address, manage and intervene with patients who express suicidal ideation or a desire to hasten death.

DEFINITIONS

DHD is the broader construct that underlies suicidal ideation, and can be used to identify cancer patients who are at risk for ending their lives. Rather than involving a wish to harm oneself, DHD

Depression and Cancer   Edited by David W. Kissane, Mario Maj and Norman Sartorius
© 2011 John Wiley & Sons, Ltd

represents a person's wish to die sooner than might occur by natural disease progression, often in the context of advanced or terminal illness.

DHD may be characterised by: (a) a passive wish (fleeting or persistent) for death without active plans; (b) a request for assistance in hastening death; or (c) an active desire and plan to commit suicide [6]. Methods for accelerating the end of life include self-injurious behaviours, euthanasia and assisted suicide [1]. Self-injurious behaviours can also include unhealthy behaviours with long-term, rather than short-term, negative consequences, which range in severity from unhealthy lifestyle choices such as smoking or non-adherence to dietary restrictions, to discontinuing potentially life-sustaining medications [1].

In cancer patients, less severe forms of suicidal ideation, such as a fleeting wish to die, are relatively common and not necessarily a cause for concern. Suicidal ideation becomes problematic when it is persistent or involves actual suicidal intent, plan, or behaviour. In these cases, a desire to act on suicidal ideation is expressed, a potential method is described, or the patient has engaged in self-injurious actions.

Physician-assisted suicide involves a physician providing the means for the patient to end his/her life, such as by prescribing a lethal dose of medication. Euthanasia is the term used when a physician administers a fatal overdose of medication with or without the patient's consent [1, 7].

PREVALENCE

Although occasional, transient thoughts of a wish to die are relatively frequent amongst cancer patients, suicidal ideation is less common [8]. In a sample of terminally ill cancer patients, 44.5% reported a fleeting desire for death, whereas only 8.5% reported a more persistent wish for hastened death [3]. A second study found that 25% of cancer patients reported that they had seriously thought about euthanasia and 12% had discussed this option with their physicians [9]. Finally, a third study identified a high DHD amongst 17% of the terminally ill patients who were assessed in a palliative care hospice setting [10].

In a 2007 review of mortality in the United States, cancer was the only physical illness significantly associated with suicide mortality [2]. Cancer patients are approximately two times more likely to commit suicide than the general population [2, 11]. At Memorial Sloan-Kettering Cancer Center, 8.6% of psychiatric consultations are suicide risk evaluation, usually provided after a patient verbally expressed suicidal ideation [12]. A study using data from the Cancer Registry of Norway [13] reported that males with cancer are 55% more likely and females with cancer are 35% more likely to die by suicide than the general population.

It is possible that the available data underestimate the true prevalence of suicidal ideation in cancer. It is difficult to estimate suicide rates, given the unknown frequency of unreported overdoses assisted by families or decisions to stop critical aspects of care such as nutrition and hydration [14]. Finally, healthcare professionals may be reluctant to report euthanasia or physician-assisted suicide to avoid possible legal and political consequences [15].

RISK OF SUICIDE IN PEOPLE WITH CANCER

In order to effectively assess and manage suicidal ideation and behaviour in cancer patients, clinicians should have a thorough understanding of the specific demographic, physical and psychosocial risk factors. A systematic review of the literature on suicide and DHD in cancer patients reported that the most common risk factors include feeling like a burden to others, loss of autonomy, a wish to control one's death, physical symptoms (e.g. severe pain), depression and hopelessness, existential concerns, lack of social support, and fear of the future [6].

Depression

The link between depression and suicide is well known in both cancer patients and the general population. Depression is a known factor in half of all suicides, and individuals suffering from depression are at a 25 times greater risk of suicide [16].

The incidence of depression is particularly high in cancer patients. About 25% of all these patients endorse severe depressive symptoms, with 6% meeting criteria for a diagnosis of major depression [3]. There is a close association between cancer and depression regardless of stage and site of disease [17]. However, patients with terminal illness are at significantly increased risk. Breitbart *et al.* [10] found that approximately 17% of patients with terminal cancer met diagnostic criteria for a major depressive episode. Depression emerged as the strongest predictor of DHD in advanced cancer patients and, amongst patients who reported significant DHD, 58% met criteria for major depression [3].

Results of an international prospective study into the association between depression and request for euthanasia in terminally ill cancer patients revealed that 44% of depressed patients requested euthanasia compared to only 15% of non-depressed patients [18]. Thus, the rate of euthanasia requests was 4.1 times greater in patients with depression. Clinicians should be aware of this relationship and continually evaluate patients to determine if depressive symptoms have reached the clinical level or are merely a reflection of appropriate feelings of sadness commonly associated with coping with a terminal diagnosis.

Hopelessness

Hopelessness was once considered under the umbrella of depressive symptoms, but has since been identified as an important construct influencing such phenomena related to end-of-life despair as DHD, suicidal ideation, and requests for assisted suicide [10, 19].

Hopelessness has been empirically linked to suicidal ideation in the general population [20, 21], with a stronger association with suicidal intent than depression [22]. A study of advanced cancer patients identified hopelessness as a stronger predictor of suicidal ideation than severity of depression [19]. Several additional studies have identified hopelessness as the strongest predictor of DHD in advanced cancer and assisted suicide [23, 24]. Breitbart *et al.* [10] concluded that hopelessness and depression were independent, significant predictors of DHD, and that the presence of both may actually be the strongest clinical marker for DHD.

Helplessness, Control and Demoralization

Suicide risk may be particularly high in cancer patients who present with an excessive need to control their lives, whereas patients who reportedly approached their medical care with acceptance and adaptability were less likely to commit suicide [25]. Personality factors such as concerns about loss of autonomy, dependency and a strong need to control the circumstances of one's death are important predictors of DHD [6].

Unfortunately, many cancer-related events such as loss of mobility, paraplegia, amputation, sensory loss, and inability to eat or swallow, can elicit feelings of helplessness, which can exacerbate these personality characteristics. Furthermore, patients may become distraught by the sense that they have lost 'control' of their minds, due to heavy sedation or episodes of delirium [26]. These symptoms can progress to what has been termed by Kissane *et al.* [27] the demoralization syndrome, which is characterised by hopelessness, loss of meaning, existential distress, a sense of incompetence, feelings of greater dependency or the perception of being a burden. In patients who present with this syndrome, the sense of impotence or helplessness can often progress to a desire to die or to commit suicide.

Lack of Social Support and Burden to Others

Well-functioning families are usually able to generate a sense of generosity and support for members with cancer, which can moderate feelings associated with DHD such as despair or demoralization. In contrast, dysfunctional families may engage in poor communication and conflict resulting in a lack of instrumental support, which is a risk factor for suicidal ideation.

Lack of social support has an established relationship to higher rates of suicide in cancer patients [28]. Several studies have found a significant correlation between lower levels of social support and a higher DHD in advanced cancer patients [3, 10, 23]. Chochinov *et al.* [3] found that poor family support was a significant predictor of DHD. Quality of social support has also been linked to reported levels of DHD [29]. Social factors, along with psychological factors, were frequently cited reasons for euthanasia requests [30].

Concerns about burdening others is significantly associated with DHD in terminally ill cancer patients [10]. A study of Oregonian patients who died by assisted suicide found that 63% of them felt that they had become a significant burden to family, friends, or other caregivers [31]. Similar perceptions of burden to others was significantly associated with DHD amongst cancer patients receiving hospice care [32]. Furthermore, in a retrospective review of terminally ill patients who committed suicide, the feeling of being a burden to others was almost universal [33].

Anxiety

Anxiety is one of the most common reasons for psychiatric consultation in terminally ill cancer patients, but has received less attention as a predictor of suicide [34]. However, a recent investigation in 200 terminally ill cancer patients revealed that high levels of anxiety were significantly related to a high level of DHD [35]. Further research in this area is needed.

Pain and Physical Symptoms

Uncontrolled pain plays an important role in vulnerability to suicide in cancer patients [14, 26, 36, 37]. Physicians have reported that persistent or uncontrolled pain fuels the majority of cancer patients' requests for assisted suicide [36]. Most cancer suicides were preceded by inadequately managed or poorly tolerated pain [25, 31, 32, 37]. Severity of pain, as well as the extent to which pain interfered with activity, significantly predicted desire for death [3, 37]. In advanced cancer patients, the presence of pain increases the likelihood of the co-occurrence of several risk factors for suicide: depression, delirium, loss of control, and hopelessness [14]. Chochinov *et al.* [3] found that

76% of patients with moderate to severe pain had significant DHD [3]. Aggressive pain management should be the first line of treatment in cases of cancer patients with DHD and suicidal ideation. DHD should then be reassessed following effective pain relief.

In addition to pain, physical symptoms also have a relationship with suicide and DHD, as they can induce psychological distress and escalate to suicidal thoughts or behaviours. Furthermore, the presence of psychological disorders may heighten perceptions of pain and other physical symptoms and contribute to suicidal thoughts. Specific physical symptoms (in particular, shortness of breath) and symptom distress have been linked to frequency of suicidal ideation [38].

Cognitive Dysfunction and Delirium

Cancer patients receiving psychiatric consultations, including assessment of suicidality, were found to have a high prevalence of organic mental disorders, primarily delirium. Estimates range from 25% to 40% [39], reaching 85% during the terminal stages of disease [40]. One third of suicidal patients receiving a psychiatric consultation at Memorial Sloan-Kettering Cancer Center were simultaneously suffering from delirium [12].

Delirium and cognitive impairment cloud a patient's reasoning ability, increasing the risk of impulsive behaviour and negatively affecting decision-making. In fact, the majority of treatment delays or refusals in cancer patients occur in the context of psychoses, organic mental disorders and/or depression, which may impair judgement [41].

History of Psychiatric Illness

Pre-existing psychiatric disturbance significantly increases the risk for DHD and suicidal ideation [42]. It is rare for a cancer patient to commit suicide without some degree of pre-morbid psychopathology [43]. Half of suicidal cancer patients receiving a psychiatric consultation at Memorial Sloan-Kettering Cancer Center had a diagnosable personality disorder. Moreover, during the psychiatric consultation, one third of these patients were also diagnosed with a major depression and half were diagnosed with an adjustment disorder with both depressed and anxious features [12]. A history of past suicide attempts or a family history of suicide also significantly increases suicide risk [14].

Physician Characteristics and Treatment Setting

Physician and treatment characteristics may influence both the degree to which patients express suicidal ideation or DHD, and how these feelings are dealt with in the context of a medical setting. Kelly *et al.* [44] identified the following factors as related to DHD in patients with terminal cancer: not being offered further treatment, lack of doctor with long-term responsibility for care, and lack of attention to psychological needs. Negative experiences with healthcare, including dissatisfaction with medical care, poor communication and lack of emotional support were also associated with higher levels of DHD [44]. A later study proposed that doctors treating terminally ill cancer patients may not be confident or well trained in eliciting psychological information and addressing suffering. Consequently, patients may withhold distress in order to protect physicians or out of fear of burdening them [45]. In a qualitative analysis based on interviews with terminally ill patients and their physicians, physicians of patients with high DHD were more likely to describe the duration of illness as long, and less likely to mention the availability of palliative care supports. Physicians' attitudes toward euthanasia, as well as their view of the patient's thoughts on euthanasia, are influential factors [46].

Researchers are increasingly concerned with the relationship between psychological distress and treatment setting [35]. Reuter *et al.* [47] reported evidence suggesting higher rates of psychological distress in cancer patients receiving inpatient care. Kelly *et al.* [32] found similar results, in that being admitted to an inpatient hospice setting was associated with DHD, along with other risk factors such as depression, perception of being a burden, low family cohesion and social support, and high levels of anxiety. A more recent study found that cancer patients receiving inpatient palliative care reported significantly higher levels of DHD than those receiving outpatient potentially life-prolonging care [35].

Demographic Characteristics of the Patient

Several patient-related factors have been associated with suicidality. Age is significantly associated with suicide risk: cancer patients in their sixties and seventies have the greatest risk [36, 48, 49]. A recent study found that suicidality was more common in patients who were previously married and had used multiple prescription drugs in the past year [50]. While men with cancer may have over twice the risk of suicide compared to the general population, the relative risk of suicide in women with cancer is less clear [13, 36, 48].

The highest suicide risk is attributed to males with respiratory cancers [3], which may also be related to the presence of other risk factors (i.e. alcohol and tobacco use) or pre-existing psychological problems. A recent study found that requests for euthanasia or assisted suicide were more common in patients with lung, pancreas, stomach, oesophagus, melanoma and head and neck cancers [51].

Stage and Trajectory of Illness

Risk of suicide may be related to cancer stage and to time since diagnosis. The first months following diagnosis is a period of great risk [13]. Additional evidence shows that cancer patients more frequently commit suicide in the advanced stages of disease, with one study reporting rates as high as 86% [25, 36, 48, 52]. Another study of cancer patients who completed suicide in Sweden found that 16% had an uncertain prognosis and 51% had a poor prognosis. Advanced cancer patients are also at increased risk for depression, pain, delirium and cognitive deficit syndromes which, as previously mentioned, may increase the likelihood of suicide [16].

Suicidal ideation and attempts are also significant in adult survivors of childhood cancer, which may be a result of physical and mental health sequelae associated with cancer treatment [53]. Additionally, breast cancer survivors, particularly black women, were found to be at increased risk for suicide for up to 25 years post treatment [54].

Spiritual and Existential Despair

Existential distress (e.g. loss of meaning, purpose, or dignity; awareness of incomplete life tasks, regret, and anxiety surrounding the existence of a higher power) are particularly relevant for cancer patients with advanced disease and may contribute to DHD [55]. DHD, hopelessness and suicidal ideation were found to be higher in terminally ill cancer patients reporting low spiritual well-being and, in particular, those who endorsed a loss of sense of meaning [56]. Terminally ill cancer patients who reported a lower sense of dignity were significantly more likely to report a loss of will to live [57]. These data suggest the critical need for the development of interventions in the terminally ill that address what many palliative care practitioners refer to as 'spiritual suffering' [58].

FACTORS THAT REDUCE SUICIDE RISK IN PEOPLE WITH CANCER

Cancer patients face considerable adversity as they cope with lifestyle changes, physical health problems and threat to life. However, not all cancer patients experience psychological distress, in fact many remain hopeful and demonstrate resilience. Resilience is defined as the ability to utilize protective factors and attain desired social, cognitive and emotional outcomes despite exposure to risk [59]. Cancer patients who had attempted suicide have significantly lower resilience scores than those who had never attempted [60].

Hope is an easily identifiable factor that enables cancer patients to be more resilient. Hope is often seen as a human strength that is not necessarily the opposite of hopelessness, and can help individuals identify meaningful and realistic desired outcomes [61]. Sullivan proposed that hope is still possible at the end of life in various forms, for cure, for survival, for comfort, for dignity, for intimacy or for salvation [62]. Level of hope is not related to cancer stage and is significantly related to coping style. Patients with high levels of hope engaged in active acceptance, normal living and reconciling with life and death [61].

LEGAL AND ETHICAL ISSUES IN ASSISTED SUICIDE

Assisted suicide remains amongst the most controversial topics in palliative care, and several important legal and ethical issues should be considered. First, this area continues to change and evolve both within the field of palliative care and the judicial system. Second, there is potential for emotionally-charged ethical dilemmas, as demonstrated by high profile media coverage of assisted suicide cases (e.g. the Dr. Jack Kevorkian and Terry Shiavo cases). Finally, the controversial nature of assisted suicide is likely to play a role in providers' assessment of and responses to patients' wishes to die, impacting subsequent treatment decisions.

The legalization of assisted suicide continues to evolve in various countries, such as Australia, where there is current debate. In Europe, forms of assisted suicide are sanctioned in the Netherlands, Belgium and Switzerland. In the United States, the issue is under the jurisdiction of each state: assisted suicide is legal in Oregon and Washington States. As a result of the 1997 Death with Dignity Act, Oregon became the first state in the United States that legalized physician-assisted suicide, permitting physicians to write prescriptions for lethal doses of medication for terminally ill residents who make this request. The U. S. Supreme Court upheld legalization with the *Gonzales* v. *Oregon* decision in 2006 [63]. In spite of the heated debate, the practice of assisted suicide by providers is still relatively rare. Since assisted suicide was legalized in Oregon, 292 patients (87% of whom had cancer) have died by this method [63]. In the Netherlands, assisted suicide and euthanasia comprise about 1–5% of all deaths and 7.4% of deaths amongst cancer patients, and these rates have remained stable over the past decade [64].

Those opposing legalization have expressed concerns that requests for assisted suicide are often due to the potentially treatable clinical correlates of DHD mentioned above [65]. Ganzini *et al.* have argued that aspects of the quality of end-of-life care, including an increase in referrals to palliative care, have improved since assisted suicide was legalized [24, 66]. Wilson *et al.* [67] recently assessed cancer patients' attitudes toward the legalization of euthanasia and physician-assisted suicide. Amongst patients receiving palliative care, the majority (59%) favoured, while only 26% firmly opposed legalization. Primary reasons for supporting legalization included the desire to have autonomy and control at the end-of-life, to avoid suffering and concerns about the futility of coping with a terminal illness.

Regardless of one's personal position on the issue of assisted suicide, comprehensive and detailed assessment of palliative care patients is critical to determine if conditions related to DHD can be modified to enhance patients' quality of life, ameliorate unnecessary suffering, and ensure that patients are not requesting assisted suicide impulsively or without a clear understanding of possible alternative solutions.

PRACTICE GUIDELINES

Assessment

The first step toward appropriate intervention in cases where there is suicide risk is careful assessment. Early and comprehensive psychiatric involvement with high-risk cancer patients can often avert suicide [68]. Healthcare professionals may be wary of conducting suicide risk assessment or responding to desire to die statements, because of fear of diminishing patients' hope, provoking emotional discussions, or the legal repercussions of possessing information about patients' suicidality [69]. However, there is no clinical research evidence to support the idea that asking about suicidal thoughts increases suicidal acts [70]. On the contrary, there is evidence that patients report a sense of relief and diminished suicidal urges once their distress and need for control over death have been acknowledged [42]. Practitioners should use assessment as a therapeutic opportunity to ask patients about their concerns about the future, provide accurate information in order to allay unwarranted fears, convey willingness to discuss these feelings, and allow patients to express feelings that may be difficult to discuss with others [71].

When patients express DHD or suicidal ideation, clinicians are immediately faced with several challenges [71]. Prior to completing any assessment, patients should be made aware of the limits of confidentiality and be advised that members of a treatment team may share patient information in an effort to provide optimal care [69]. It is crucial to assess the patient's intended meaning and underlying cause of the suicidal ideation or DHD statements quickly. Healthcare professionals should be aware of and evaluate the risk factors associated with DHD that were reviewed above (e.g. depression and severe pain) through the use of detailed interviews and standardized measures.

Specific recommendations and guidelines have been developed to assist practitioners with challenging discussions about this sensitive topic (Table 6.1) [6]. The goal of the guidelines is to offer pragmatic solutions and ensure that these discussions are less difficult, more effective, and address the most salient issues. These guidelines are flexible and should be implemented over time and within the context of a trusting relationship [71]. A therapeutic response to DHD includes empathy, active listening, management of realistic expectations, permission to discuss psychological distress, and the provision of a referral to other professionals when appropriate (Table 6.2). Systematic reviews of randomized, controlled trials have shown that this approach ameliorates distress and promotes psychological well-being [70].

Comprehensive evaluations of the severity and intensity of suicidal ideation will then help to inform appropriate intervention and treatment planning. According to Rudd and Joiner [72], the following factors should be evaluated to identify those individuals who are at highest risk for suicidal behaviour: predisposition to this behaviour (i.e., a history of suicidal behaviour, psychiatric diagnosis, and demographic risk factors); precipitants or stressors; symptomatic presentation (i.e., depression, anger and agitation); nature of suicidal thinking (frequency, intensity, duration, specificity of plans, availability of means, and explicitness of intent); hopelessness; nature of previous attempts (frequency, method, lethality and outcome); impulsivity and lack of protective factors (social and family support, problem-solving skills, and mental health treatment). Additionally, evaluation of palliative care patients requires careful assessment of somatic symptoms to determine whether their aetiology is psychiatric or organic in nature [8, 73].

Hudson *et al.* [71] developed a two-phased approach for how healthcare providers should respond to patients' desire to die statements. Phase I involves assessment and exploration of the expression

Table 6.1 General guidelines for the assessment of suicide and desire for hastened death in patients with cancer (adapted from National Breast Cancer Center and National Cancer Control Initiative [70] and Hudson et al. [71])

Be alert to your own responses	• Be aware of how your responses influence discussions • Monitor your attitude and responses • Demonstrate positive regard for the patient • Seek supervision
Be open to hearing concerns	• Gently ask about emotional concerns • Be alert to verbal and non-verbal distress cues • Encourage expression of feelings • Actively listen, without interrupting • Discuss desire for death using patient's words • Permit sadness, silence and tears • Express empathy verbally and non-verbally • Acknowledge differences in responses to illness
Assess contributing factors	• Prior psychiatric history • Prior suicide attempts • History of alcohol or substance abuse • Lack of social support • Feelings of burden • Family conflict • Need for additional assistance • Depression and anxiety • Existential concerns, loss of meaning and dignity • Cognitive impairment • Physical symptoms, especially severe pain
Respond to specific issues	• Acknowledge patient or family fears and concerns • Address modifiable contributing factors • Recommend interventions • Develop plan to manage more complicated issues
Conclude discussion	• Summarize and review important points • Clarify patient perceptions

	• Provide opportunity for questions
	• Assist in facilitating discussion with others
	• Provide appropriate referrals
After discussion	• Document discussion in medical records
	• Communicate with members of the treatment team

Table 6.2 Questions to ask patients and family when assessing suicidal risk (adapted from Holland *et al.* [80])

Acknowledge that these are common thoughts that can be discussed	• Most patients with cancer have passing thoughts about suicide, such as 'I might do something if it gets bad enough'. Have you ever had thoughts like that? • Have you had any thoughts of not wanting to live? • Have you had those thoughts in the past few days?
Assess level of risk	• Do you have thoughts about wanting to end your life? How? • Do you have a plan? • Do you have any strong social supports? • Do you have pills stockpiled at home? • Do you own or have access to a weapon?
Obtain prior history	• Have you ever had a psychiatric disorder, suffered from depression, or made a suicide attempt? • Is there a family history of suicide?
Identify substance abuse	• Have you had a problem with alcohol or drugs?
Identify bereavement	• Have you lost anyone close to you recently?
Identify medical predictors of risk	• Do you have pain that is not being relieved? • How has the disease affected your life? • How is your memory and concentration? • Do you feel hopeless? • What do you plan for the future?

of DHD to foster a better understanding of underlying factors. In this phase, it is important to assess the nature of a desire to die statement by focusing on a patient's current feelings and fears, as well as assessing the patient's suffering across physical, spiritual, psychosocial and existential domains. Phase II involves evaluation of factors that may be contributing to the patient's desire to die, again by focusing on the patient's current feelings and fears, and by assessing his or her suffering across the previously mentioned domains. This information can help clinicians with preliminary interventions or to make appropriate referrals to professionals with specific expertise (e.g. to a mental health professional, pastoral care, or palliative care).

Instruments for the Assessment of Risk of Suicide and DHD

In order to improve assessment methods and gain a better understanding of the complex construct of DHD, researchers have developed specific scales. These measures include the Desire for Death Rating Scale (DDRS) [3], the Schedule of Attitudes toward Hastened Death (SAHD) [74, 75], the Beck Hopelessness Scale [21, 76] and the Demoralization Scale [77] and have been validated in populations with advanced disease.

Specific measures of suicidality that are appropriate for use in medically ill populations include the Beck Scale for Suicidal Ideation [78] and the Modified Scale for Suicidal Ideation [79]. They assess duration and frequency of ideation, sense of control over making an attempt, deterrents, and amount of actual preparation. Standardized measures utilized in a sensitive manner, within the context of a trusting patient-provider relationship, can help clinicians to identify patients' needs and to appropriately tailor interventions.

Intervention Strategies

Competent interventions for suicide may provide cancer patients with great relief from distress and suffering and ultimately save lives. When implementing interventions, regardless of technique and modality,

Table 6.3 Interventions for the suicidal patient (adapted Holland *et al.* [80])

For patients whose suicidal threat are seen as serious	• Provide constant observation and further assessment • Dangerous objects like guns or potentially lethal medications should be removed from the room or home. • The risk for suicidal behaviour should be communicated to family members.
For the patients who are not acutely suicidal and is medically stable	• Patient should agree to call when feeling overwhelmed, making a contract with the physician to talk about suicidal thoughts in the future rather than to act on them.
For inpatients	• Room searches should be carried out to make sure there are no means available for self-destructive behaviour. • The patient should be under constant observation from the time suicidal thoughts are expressed.
For severely suicidal outpatients whose suicidal thoughts are not acutely caused by their medical condition or medication	• Psychiatric hospitalization is warranted, either by voluntary or involuntary means. • A psychiatrist can assist in making these arrangements. Document medical action and reasoning in the crisis.

practitioners must assess risk factors for suicide, as discussed above.

Initial interventions should focus on determining imminent risk and making necessary plans and arrangements for patient safety (Table 6.3). Appropriate interventions may include psychiatric hospitalization for severely suicidal patients, the use of suicide prevention resources, contracting with the patient for safety, limiting access to potential means such as pills or guns, involvement of family or friends in monitoring the patient, and referral to experts as needed [80]. However, it should be noted that psychiatric hospitalization may not be ideal or realistic for severely medically ill patients. Crisis intervention and the mobilization of support systems may act as external controls and strongly reduce the risk of suicide [26].

The second level of interventions should utilize specific risk factors to inform targeted intervention strategies that may reduce suicidality, such as the aggressive management of pain, physical symptoms, delirium and cognitive impairment [42]. Antidepressant medications in tandem with supportive psychotherapy, cognitive-behavioural techniques, and patient and family education are the most effective means for improving depressive symptoms, hopelessness and suicidal ideation [81, 82]. Additional pharmacological interventions should be used to treat symptoms of depression and any accompanying symptoms of anxiety, agitation, psychosis, or pain [6, 8]. A recent study demonstrated that desire for death was often ameliorated when depression was resolved in response to treatment with antidepressant medication [83].

Cognitive-behavioural techniques can be tailored to manage cancer patients' physical symptoms and challenge cognitive distortions driving suicidal ideation and hopelessness [84–86]. Both individual and group supportive psychotherapy for cancer patients can provide additional support by assuaging feelings of isolation, bolstering coping skills, and addressing existential concerns [55, 80, 87]. Conversations about advanced care directives have the potential to facilitate discussion of end-of-life issues and concerns amongst patients and their families [8, 88]. Additionally, if patients are feeling burdensome to caregivers, facilitating communication about their relationships may be helpful [6].

Interventions focused on enhancing patients' sense of meaning [89, 90], dignity [57, 91] and responding to spiritual and existential concerns have much to offer. An intervention based on mindfulness theory, teaching patients to focus on the moment, may help to alleviate distress and fears about the future [92]. Mindfulness techniques, combined with behavioural techniques and emotion regulation, often used in interventions like dialectical behaviour therapy to manage suicidal behaviour, may be effective with cancer patients as well.

RESEARCH CHALLENGES AND OPPORTUNITIES

There are numerous methodological limitations specific to research on DHD and suicide in cancer. There is a call for more longitudinal research to accurately assess the dynamic and fleeting nature of DHD. Overall, our knowledge of the construct is limited and could be more accurately assessed through multiple assessments. However, longitudinal studies may be taxing on terminally ill patients, who are most vulnerable to DHD and suicidal ideation. More research is needed on patients currently experiencing DHD [6]. Assessments in families are often conducted after the patient's death, and may be influenced by grief and the general effect of time. Future research opportunities include further investigation of additional potential predictors of DHD such as demographic and cultural variables, personality factors, social support, cognitive impairment, need for a sense of control, and spiritual concerns [6]. Finally, more attention is needed to the development of interventions to prevent and treat DHD with the goal of alleviating suffering at the end of life.

CONCLUSIONS

The management of suicidality and DHD in cancer patients raises clinical, legal, ethical and moral issues for healthcare professionals, and involves not only the medical arena but also the legal system. In addition, there are a multitude of complex risk factors that may contribute to the manifestation of DHD or suicidality, which are only partially studied. Currently available guidelines for the assessment and management of DHD and suicidality, and the ability to deliver empirically-supported psychosocial and pharmacological interventions, should assist healthcare providers to meet these challenges and result in better outcomes for patients.

REFERENCES

1. Mishara, B.L. (1999) Synthesis of research and evidence on factors affecting the desire of terminally ill or seriously chronically ill persons to hasten death. *Omega*, **39,** 1–70.
2. Rockett, I.R., Wang, S., Lian, Y. and Stack, S. (2007) Suicide-associated comorbidity among US males and females: a multiple cause-of-death analysis. *Inj. Prev.*, **13,** 311–315.

3. Chochinov, H.M., Wilson, K.G., Enns, M. *et al.* (1995) Desire for death in the terminally ill. *Am. J. Psychiatry*, **152,** 1185–1191.

4. Olden, M., Pessin, H., Lictenthal, W.G. and Breitbart, W. (2009) Suicide and desire for hastened death in the terminally ill, in *Handbook of Psychiatry in Palliative Medicine* (eds. H.M. Chochinov and W. Breitbart), Oxford University Press, New York, pp. 101–112.

5. Pessin, H., Amakawa, L. and Breitbart, W. (2010) Suicide, in *Psycho-Oncology*, 2nd edn (ed. J. Holland), Oxford University Press, New York, pp. 319–323.

6. Hudson, P.L., Kristjanson, L.J., Ashby, M. *et al.* (2006) Desire for hastened death in patients with advanced disease and the evidence base of clinical guidelines: a systematic review. *Palliative Med.*, **20,** 693–701.

7. Cohen, J.S., Fihn, S.D., Boyko, E.J. *et al.* (1994) Attitudes toward assisted suicide and euthanasia among physicians in Washington State. *N. Engl. J. Med.*, **331,** 89–94.

8. Pessin, H., Potash, M. and Breitbart, W. (2003) Diagnosis, assessment, and treatment of depression in palliative care, in *Psychosocial Issues in Palliative Care* (ed. M. Lloyd-Williams), Oxford University Press, Oxford, pp. 81–103.

9. Emanuel, E.J., Fairclough, D.L., Daniels, E.R. and Clarridge, B.R. (1996) Euthanasia and physician-assisted suicide: a comparative study of physicians, terminally-ill cancer patients, and the general population. *Lancet*, **347,** 1805–1810.

10. Breitbart, W., Rosenfeld, B., Pessin, H. *et al.* (2000) Depression, hopelessness, and desire for hastened death in terminally ill patients with cancer. *JAMA*, **284,** 2907–2911.

11. Levi, F., Bulliard, J.L. and La Vecchia, C. (1990) Suicide risk among incident cases of cancer in the Swiss Canton of Vaud. *Oncology*, **48,** 44–47.

12. Breitbart, W. (1987) Suicide in cancer patients. *Oncology*, **1,** 49–55.

13. Hem, E., Loge, J.H., Haldorsen, T. and Ekeberg, O. (2004) Suicide risk in cancer patients from 1960 to 1999. *J. Clin. Oncol.*, **22,** 4209–4216.

14. Breitbart, W. (1993) Suicide risk and pain in cancer and AIDS patients, in *Current and Emerging Issues in Cancer Pain: Research and Practice* (eds. C.R. Chapman and K.M. Foley), Raven Press, New York, pp. 49–65.

15. Rosenfeld, B. (2000) Methodological issues in assisted suicide and euthanasia research. *Psychol. Public Policy Law*, **6,** 559–574.

16. Breitbart, W., Gibson, C., Abbey, J. *et al.* (2006) Suicide in palliative care, in *Textbook of Palliative Medicine* (eds. E. Bruera, I.

J. Higginson, C. Ripamonti and C. Von Guten), Hodder Arnold, London, pp. 860–868.

17. Massie, M.J. (2004) Prevalence of depression in patients with cancer. *J. Natl. Cancer Inst. Monogr.*, **32**, 57–71.

18. van der Lee, M.L., van der Bom, J.G., Swarte, N.B. *et al.* (2005) Euthanasia and depression: a prospective cohort study among terminally ill cancer patients. *J. Clin. Oncol.*, **23**, 1–6.

19. Chochinov, H.M., Wilson, K.G., Enns, M. and Lander, S. (1998) Depression, hopelessness, and suicidal ideation in the terminally ill. *Psychosomatics*, **39**, 366–370.

20. Minkoff, K., Bergman, E., Beck, A.T. and Beck, R. (1973) Hopelessness, depression, and attempted suicide. *Am. J. Psychiatry*, **130**, 455–459.

21. Beck, A.T., Kovacs, M. and Weissman, A. (1975) Hopelessness and suicidal behavior. An overview. *JAMA*, **234**, 1146–1149.

22. Wetzel, R.D. (1976) Hopelessness, depression, and suicide intent. *Arch. Gen. Psychiatry*, **33**, 1069–1073.

23. Rodin, G., Zimmermann, C., Rydall, A. *et al.* (2007) The desire for hastened death in patients with metastatic cancer. *J. Pain Symptom Manag.*, **33**, 661–675.

24. Ganzini, L., Nelson, H.D., Lee, M.A. *et al.* (2001) Oregon physicians' attitudes about and experiences with end-of-life care since passage of the Oregon Death with Dignity Act. *JAMA*, **285**, 2363–2369.

25. Farberow, N.L., Schneiderman, E.S. and Leonard, C.V. (1963) Suicide among general medical and surgical hospital patients with malignant neoplasms. *Med. Bull. Veterans Admin.*, **9**, 1–11.

26. Breitbart, W., Gibson, C., Abbey, J. and Iannarone, N. (2006) Suicide in palliative care, in *Textbook of Palliative Medicine* (eds. E. Bruera, I.J. Higginson, C. Ripamonti and C. von Gunten), Hodder Arnold, London, pp. 860–868.

27. Kissane, D.W., Clarke, D.M. and Street, A.F. (2001) Demoralization syndrome - a relevant psychiatric diagnosis for palliative care. *J. Palliat. Care*, **17**, 12–21.

28. Abbey, J. G. (2008) Communication about end-of-life topics between terminally ill cancer patients and their family members. January 1, 2008. ETD Collection for Fordham University. Paper AAI3337626.

29. Rosenfeld, B., Krivo, S., Breitbart, W. and Chochinov, H.M. (2000) Suicide, assisted suicide, and euthanasia in the terminally ill, in *Handbook of Psychiatry in Palliative Medicine* (eds. H.M. Chochinov and W. Breitbart), Oxford University Press, New York, pp. 51–62.

30. van der Maas, P.J., van der Wal, G., Haverkate, I. *et al.* (1996) Euthanasia, physician-assisted suicide, and other medical practices involving the end of life in the Netherlands, 1990–1995. *N. Engl. J. Med.*, **335**, 1699–1705.

31. Sullivan, A.D., Hedberg, K. and Hopkins, D. (2001) Legalized physician-assisted suicide in Oregon, 1998–2000. *N. Engl. J. Med.*, **344**, 605–607.

32. Kelly, B., Burnett, P., Pelusi, D. *et al.* (2003) Factors associated with the wish to hasten death: a study of patients with terminal illness. *Psychol. Med.*, **33**, 75–81.

33. Street, A. and Kissane, D. (1999–2000) Dispensing death, desiring death: an exploration of medical roles and patient motivation during the period of legalized euthanasia in Australia. *Omega*, **40**, 272–280.

34. Wilson, K.G., Chochinov, H.M., Skirko, M.G. *et al.* (2007) Depression and anxiety disorders in palliative cancer care. *J. Pain Symptom Manag.*, **33**, 118–129.

35. Kolva, E., Rosenfeld, B., Pessin, H. *et al.* (2010) *Anxiety in Terminally Ill Cancer Patients: Palliative vs. Life-Prolonging Care*, Society for Behavioral Medicine, Seattle.

36. Bolund, C. (1985) Suicide and cancer II. Medical and care factors in suicide by cancer patients in Sweden, 1973–1976. *J. Psychosoc. Oncol.*, **3**, 31–52.

37. Mystakidou, K., Parpa, E., Katsouda, E. *et al.* (2005) Pain and desire for hastened death in terminally ill cancer patients. *Cancer Nurs.*, **28**, 318–324.

38. Suarez-Almazor, M.E., Newman, C., Hanson, J. and Bruera, E. (2002) Attitudes of terminally ill cancer patients about euthanasia and assisted suicide: predominance of psychosocial determinants and beliefs over symptoms distress and subsequent survival. *J. Clin. Oncol.*, **20**, 2134–2141.

39. Pessin, H., Rosenfeld, B., Burton, L. and Breitbart, W. (2003) The role of cognitive impairment in desire for hastened death: a study of patients with advanced AIDS. *Gen. Hosp. Psychiat.*, **25**, 194–199.

40. Massie, M.J., Holland, J. and Glass, E. (1983) Delirium in terminally ill cancer patients. *Am. J. Psychiatry*, **140**, 1048–1050.

41. Filiberti, A. and Ripamonti, C. (2002) Suicide and suicidal thoughts in cancer patients. *Tumori*, **88**, 193–199.

42. Pessin, H., Evcimen, Y.A., Apostolatos, A. and Breitbart, W. (2008) Diagnosis, assessment, and treatment of depression in palliative care, in

Psychosocial Issues in Palliative Care (ed. M. Lloyd-Williams), Oxford University Press, New York, pp. 129–159.

43. Holland, J.C. (1982) Psychological aspects of cancer, in *Cancer Medicine*, 2nd edn (eds. J. Holland and E. Frei), Lea & Febiger, Philadelphia, pp. 1175–1203.

44. Kelly, B., Burnett, P., Pelusi, D. *et al.* (2002) Terminally ill cancer patients wish to hasten death. *Palliative Med.*, **16,** 339–345.

45. Kelly, B., Pelusi, D., Burnett, P. and Varghese, F. (2004) The prevalence of psychiatric disorder and the wish to hasten death among terminally ill cancer patients. *Palliat. Support. Care*, **2,** 163–169.

46. Kelly, B., Burnett, P., Pelusi, D. *et al.* (2003) Doctors and their patients: a context for understanding the wish to hasten death. *Psychooncology*, **12,** 375–384.

47. Reuter, K., Raugust, S., Marschiner, N. and Harter, M. (2007) Differences in prevalence rates of psychological distress and mental disorders in inpatients and outpatients with breast and gynaecological cancer. *Eu. J. Cancer Care*, **16,** 222–230.

48. Bolund, C. (1985) Suicide and cancer I. Demographic and social characteristics of cancer patients who committed suicide in Sweden, 1973–1976. *J. Psychosoc. Oncol.*, **3,** 17–30.

49. Hietanen, P., Lönnqvist, J., Henriksson, M. and Jallinoja, P. (1994) Do cancer suicides differ from others? *Psychooncology*, **3,** 189–195.

50. Schneider, K. and Shenassa, E. (2008) Correlates of suicide ideation in a population-based sample of cancer patients. *J. Psychosoc. Oncol.*, **26,** 49–62.

51. Abarshi, E., Onwuteaka-Philipsen, B. and van der Wal, G. (2009) Euthanasia requests and cancer types in the Netherlands: is there a relationship? *Health Policy*, **89,** 168–173.

52. Ransom, S., Sacco, W.P., Weitzner, M.A. *et al.* (2006) Interpersonal factors predict increased desire for hastened death in late-stage cancer patients. *Ann. Behav. Med.*, **31,** 63–69.

53. Recklitis, C.J., Lockwood, R.A., Rothwell, M.A. and Diller, L.R. (2006) Suicidal ideation and attempts in adult survivors of childhood cancer. *J. Clin. Oncol.*, **24,** 3852–3857.

54. Schairer, C., Brown, L.M., Chen, B.E. *et al.* (2006) Suicide after breast cancer: an international population-based study of 723 810 women. *J. Natl. Cancer Inst.*, **98,** 1416–1419.

55. Breitbart, W. (2002) Spirituality and meaning in supportive care: spirituality- and meaning-centered group psychotherapy interventions in advanced cancer. *Support Care Cancer*, **10,** 272–280.

56. McClain, C.S., Rosenfeld, B. and Breitbart, W. (2003) Effect of spiritual well-being on end-of-life despair in terminally-ill cancer patients. *Lancet*, **361**, 1603–1607.

57. Chochinov, H.M. (2002) Dignity-conserving care – a new model for palliative care: helping the patient feel valued. *JAMA*, **287**, 2253–2260.

58. Rousseau, P. (2000) Spirituality and the dying patient. *J. Clin. Oncol.*, **18**, 2000–2002.

59. Betancourt, T.S. and Khan, K.T. (2008) The mental health of children affected by armed conflict: protective processes and pathways to resilience. *Int. Rev. Psychiatry*, **20**, 317–328.

60. Roy, A., Sarchiapone, M. and Carli, V. (2007) Low resilience in suicide attempters. *Arch. Suicide Res.*, **11**, 265–269.

61. Chi, G.C. (2007) The role of hope in patients with cancer. *Oncol. Nurs. Forum*, **34**, 415–421.

62. Sullivan, M.D. (2003) Hope and hopelessness at the end of life. *Am. J. Geriatr. Psychiatry*, **11**, 393–405.

63. Oregon Department of Health Services (2007) *Death with Dignity Act Annual Report 2006*, Oregon Department of Health Services, Salem.

64. Onwuteaka-Philipsen, B.D., van der Heide, A., Koper, D. *et al.* (2003) Euthanasia and other end-of-life decisions in the Netherlands in 1990, 1995, and 2001. *Lancet*, **362**, 395–399.

65. Okie, S. (2005) Physician-assisted suicide - Oregon and beyond. *N. Engl. J. Med.*, **352**, 1627–1630.

66. National Health and Medical Research Council Australia (2003) *Clinical Practice Guidelines for the Psychosocial Care of Adults with Cancer*, National Health and Medical Research Council Australia, Canberra.

67. Wilson, K.G., Chochinov, H.M., McPherson, C.J. *et al.* (2007) Desire for euthanasia or physician-assisted suicide in palliative cancer care. *Health Psychol.*, **26**, 314–323.

68. Dubovsky, S.L. (1978) Averting suicide in terminally ill patients. *Psychosomatics*, **19**, 113–115.

69. Schwartz, J.K. (2003) Understanding and responding to patients' requests for assistance in dying. *J. Nurs. Scholarship*, **35**, 377–384.

70. National Breast Cancer Center and National Cancer Control Initiative (2003) *Clinical Practice Guidelines for the Psychosocial Care of Adults with Cancer*, National Breast Cancer Center, Camperdown.

71. Hudson, P.L., Schofield, P., Kelly, B. *et al.* (2006) Responding to desire to die statements from patients with advanced disease: recommendations for health professionals. *Palliative Med.*, **200**, 703–710.

72. Rudd, M.D. and Joiner, T. (1999) Assessment of suicidality in outpatient practice, in *Innovation in Clinical Practice: A Sourcebook* (eds. L. VandeCreek and R. Jackson), Professional Resource Press, Sarasota, pp. 101–117.

73. Pessin, H., Olden, M., Jacobson, C. and Kosinski, A. (2005) Clinical assessment of depression in terminally ill cancer patients: a practical guide. *Palliat. Support Care*, **3**, 319–324.

74. Rosenfeld, B., Breitbart, W., Galietta, M. *et al.* (2000) The schedule of attitudes toward hastened death: measuring desire for death in terminally ill cancer patients. *Cancer*, **88**, 2868–2875.

75. Rosenfeld, B., Breitbart, W., Stein, K. *et al.* (1999) Measuring desire for death among patients with HIV/AIDS: the schedule of attitudes toward hastened death. *Am. J. Psychiatry*, **156**, 94–100.

76. Abbey, J.G., Rosenfeld, B., Pessin, H. and Breitbart, W. (2006) Hopelessness at the end of life: the utility of the Hopelessness Scale with terminally ill cancer patients. *Br. J. Health Psychol.*, **11**, 173–183.

77. Kissane, D.W., Wein, S., Love, A. *et al.* (2004) The Demoralization Scale: a report of its development and preliminary validation. *J. Palliative Care*, **20**, 269–276.

78. Beck, A.T. and Steer, R.A. (1991) *Manual for Beck Scale for Suicidal Ideation*, Pennsylvania Corporation, New York.

79. Miller, I.W., Norman, W.H., Bishop, S.B. and Dow, M.G. (1986) The Modified Scale for Suicidal Ideation: reliability and validity. *J. Consult. Clin. Psychol.*, **54**, 724–725.

80. Holland, J., Greenberg, D. and Hughes, M. (eds.) (2006) *Quick Reference for Oncology Clinicians. The Psychiatric and Psychological Dimensions of Cancer Symptom Management*, IPOS Press, Charlottesville.

81. Maguire, P., Hopwood, P., Tarrier, N. and Howell, T. (1985) Treatment of depression in cancer patients. *Acta Psychiatr. Scand.*, **320** (Suppl.), 81–84.

82. Block, S.D. (2006) Psychological issues in end-of-life care. *J. Palliat. Med.*, **9**, 751–772.

83. Breitbart, W., Rosenfeld, B., Gibson, C. *et al.* (2010) Impact of treatment for depression on desire for hastened death in patients with advanced AIDS. *Psychosomatics*, **51**, 98–105.

84. Moorey, S. and Greer, S. (2002) *Cognitive Behaviour Therapy for People with Cancer*, Oxford University Press, New York.
85. Tatrow, K. and Montgomery, G.H. (2006) Cognitive behavioral therapy techniques for distress and pain in breast cancer patients: a meta-analysis. *J. Behav. Med.*, **29**, 17–27.
86. Massie, M.J. and Holland, J.C. (1990) Depression and the cancer patient. *J. Clin. Psychiatry*, **51** (Suppl.), 12–17.
87. Spiegel, D., Bloom, J.R. and Yalom, I. (1981) Group support for patients with metastatic cancer. A randomized outcome study. *Arch. Gen. Psychiatry*, **38**, 527–533.
88. Menon, A.S., Campbell, D., Ruskin, P. and Hebel, J.R. (2000) Depression, hopelessness, and the desire for life-saving treatments among eldery medically ill veterans. *Am. J. Geriatr. Psychiatry*, **8**, 333–342.
89. Breitbart, W. (2003) Reframing hope: meaning-centered care for patients near the end of life. *J. Palliat. Med.*, **6**, 979–88.
90. Breitbart, W., Gibson, C., Poppito, S.R. and Berg, A. (2004) Psychotherapeutic interventions at the end of life: a focus on meaning and spirituality. *Can. J. Psychiatry*, **49**, 366–372.
91. Chochinov, H.M., Hack, T., Hassard, T. *et al.* (2005) Dignity therapy: a novel psychotherapeutic intervention for patients near the end of life. *J. Clin. Oncol.*, **23**, 5520–5525.
92. Smith, J., Richardson, J., Hoffman, C. and Pilkington, K. (2005) Mindfulness-based stress reduction as supportive therapy in cancer care: systematic review. *J. Adv. Nurs.*, **52**, 315–327.

CHAPTER 7

Pharmacotherapy of Depression in People with Cancer

Luigi Grassi and Maria Giulia Nanni
Section of Psychiatry, Department of Medical Sciences of Communication and Behaviour, University of Ferrara, Italy

Yosuke Uchitomi
Department of Neuropsychiatry, Okayama University, Okayama, Japan

Michelle Riba
Department of Psychiatry, University of Michigan, Ann Arbor, MI, USA

Over the last twenty years, attention has increasingly turned to the problem of depression amongst cancer patients [1, 2]. The incidence of depression in cancer has been shown to range from 4.5 to 58%, with percentages varying according to diagnosis (major depression, dysthymia, adjustment disorder with depressed mood), gender, age, site of cancer and clinical setting (ambulatory, inpatient oncology units, palliative care) [3]. The consequences of depression for cancer patients are remarkable, with several studies indicating a significant relationship between depression and reduction of the patient's quality

Depression and Cancer   Edited by David W. Kissane, Mario Maj and Norman Sartorius
© 2011 John Wiley & Sons, Ltd

of life, increase in the subjective perception of pain, desire for hastened death and suicidal ideation, decreased adherence to treatment, prolonged length of hospital stay, increased family distress and worse prognosis [4].

In spite of these data, several barriers still exist in properly screening, diagnosing and treating depression in oncology settings. As reported by Greenberg [5], cultural, organizational and specific issues continue to represent a problem in the delivery of mental health interventions in medical settings: e.g. a very low proportion of patients discuss their low mood with their doctors; oncologists use to address clinical issues such as pain, but not affective symptoms and depression; mental health departments commonly have difficulty in developing programs for cancer patients; and mental health specialists often work in systems that are isolated, or 'siloed' from oncologists. Amongst elderly people, in whom the incidence of both depression and cancer is higher, the problems are even more significant [6].

For these reasons, a more sensitive, collaborative and comprehensive approach to the diagnosis and treatment of depression, including clinical education, enhanced role of nurses, and integrating oncology and specialist care, is recommended in the clinical setting [7]. Some steps forward have been taken in favouring routine evaluation of depression through the application of reliable tools in oncology settings and the development of specific educational models, such as the National Comprehensive Cancer Network Distress Management guidelines [8]. Standardized charting of distress as the sixth vital sign would help earlier recognition [9]. However, screening and diagnosing is not enough, since a number of studies have indicated that even when cancer patients are diagnosed with major depression, only one-third receive any antidepressant medication, very few take a therapeutic dose for an adequate period and very few receive psychological treatment or are referred to mental health services [10–12]. Even when referred to mental health services, a very low proportion (25–30%) of cancer patients with depression accept this referral and therefore very few receive proper psychopharmacological intervention [13].

Amongst cancer patients in an advanced phase of illness, the situation is even worse. The diagnosis and treatment of depression in palliative care cancer patients represents a major challenge for psychiatry [14]. The symptoms of lethargy, poor appetite, sleep disruption and fatigue may easily be attributed to cancer and its treatment, rather than depression; the depressive state may be frequently interpreted as a physiological and understandable reaction to the severity of the patient's physical condition or the imminence of death; the patient's short survival time may make it impossible to achieve a significant response to treatment [15].

While the use of antidepressants (ADs) in cancer patients has increased in the last 20–25 years [16–18], this does not necessarily correspond to an improved treatment of depression or acknowledgement of the importance of the problem. ADs are also prescribed for hot flushes, nausea and pain, and the relationship between increased prescription of ADs and outcomes of depression care in cancer is unclear at this time [19, 20].

Thus, although cancer increases the need for mental health services [21], cancer patients with depression have a low rate of utilization of these services [22]. It is mandatory that healthcare professionals working in oncology, such as oncologists, surgeons, radiation oncologists, general practitioners, nurses, social workers and psychologists, receive training in psychiatry. Recent consensus guidelines, algorithms and reviews advocate the need to correctly assess and treat depression in cancer and have been developed and proposed in the hope to promote an integrated psychopharmacological and psychosocial treatment [23, 24].

In this chapter, we focus on the pharmacological treatment of depression in cancer patients by examining the clinical use of ADs and their interaction with chemotherapy and anticancer agents. We also discuss the literature showing the possible benefits of the 'off label' use of certain ADs for cancer-related symptoms (e.g. pain, hot flushes, fatigue).

CLINICAL USE OF ANTIDEPRESSANTS IN THE TREATMENT OF DEPRESSION IN PATIENTS WITH CANCER

A series of open-label and clinical case studies about the use of ADs in patients with cancer have been published over the years, providing the clinician with useful information about the dosage, efficacy and side effects of these drugs. Only a few placebo-controlled double-blind randomized trials have been conducted [25]. This may be explained by the difficulty to fulfil the usual inclusion and exclusion criteria of randomized controlled trials in patients with cancer. For instance, cancer patients receive many different types of drugs, their clinical status may prevent them from participating in trials, and ethical concerns may exist, especially in palliative care patients.

The main characteristics of ADs are summarized in Table 7.1. The first ADs have been available for more than 50 years: they include tricyclics (TCAs), such as amitriptyline and imipramine, and monoamine oxidase inhibitors (MAOIs), such as phenelzine. However, it is the development of newer ADs over the last 20 years that has substantially modified the approach to depression in cancer patients: they include selective serotonin reuptake inhibitors (SSRIs), such as sertraline and citalopram, and selective noradrenaline and serotonin reuptake inhibitors (SNRIs), such as venlafaxine and duloxetine.

A good knowledge of and careful attention to the profile of the ADs and their side effects are extremely important when using these drugs in oncology. Patients with cancer often have problems with constipation, urinary retention, seizures, stomatitis, or cardiac problems such as orthostatic hypotension and arrhythmias, requiring careful selection of the AD.

The use of MAOIs is generally contraindicated and not considered safe in cancer patients, because of the high risk of side effects. MAOIs can interact with opioids, sympathomimetics and procarbazine and cause severe hypertensive crises. In addition, MAOIs interact with some anaesthetic drugs during surgery and patients with cancer often undergo surgical procedures.

The use of TCAs has been gradually decreasing, mainly because their antimuscarinic properties may be extremely negative or even dangerous for cancer patients (e.g. dry mouth in patients with mucositis due to chemotherapy, worsening of reduction of bowel peristalsis in patients receiving opioids for pain, possible confusional states and delirium in debilitated cancer patients).

In contrast, the use of SSRIs and SNRIs has increased as a result of their higher safety profile [26, 27], although some precautions

Table 7.1 Antidepressant medications and their use in cancer patients

Class	Action	Side effects Possible disadvantages	Side effects Possible advantages	Use in cancer patients
Trycyclic antidepressants (e.g. amitriptyline, imipramine, desipramine, clomipramine)	Inhibition of 5-HT and NA reuptake		Action on pain	Generally not used for the risky antimuscarinic side effects. If necessary, use with caution
	Antimuscarinic	Constipation, dry mouth, urinary retention, memory dysfunction		
	Antihistaminic	Drowsiness	Action on sleep	
	Anti alpha1	Postural hypotension, dizziness, reflex tachycardia		
		Hypotension		
Selective serotonin reuptake inhibitors (fluoxetine, fluvoxamine, paroxetine, sertraline, citalopram, escitalopram)	Inhibition of 5-HT reuptake	Sexual dysfunction (5-HT2A)	Some more sedative (e.g. citalopram) than others	Regularly used, with the exception of fluvoxamine (high interaction with CYP). Paroxetine reported to interfere with tamoxifen
		Gastrointestinal effects (nausea, vomiting, diarrhoea) (5HT3)		
Selective noradrenaline reuptake inhibitors (e.g. reboxetine)	Inhibition of NA reuptake	Decreased blood pressure, dizziness	Improved drive and cognitive functions	Not routinely used
	Slight antimuscarinic	Possible dry mouth, urinary retention		
Selective serotonin and noradrenaline reuptake inhibitors (e.g. venlafaxine, desvenlafaxine, duloxetine, milnacipram)	Inhibition of 5-HT and NA reuptake	Possible risk of hypertension	Action on pain	More frequently used

(continued)

Table 7.1 (*continued*)

Class	Action	Side effects Possible disadvantages	Side effects Possible advantages	Use in cancer patients
Selective dopamine and noradrenaline reuptake inhibitors (e.g. buproprion)	Inhibition of dopamine and NA reuptake	Anxiety Psychomotor activation	Increase attention and concentration Possibly decrease fatigue	Some data on patients with fatigue or in an advanced phase. Check risk of seizures
Noradrenergic and specific serotonergic antidepressants (e.g. mirtazapine)	Increase 5-HT and NA activity		Increase appetite and weight gain	More frequently used. Check possible (rare) neutropenia
	Antihistaminic	Drowsiness	Drowsiness (helpful in case of insomnia)	
Serotonin antagonists and reuptake inhibitors (trazodone, nefazodone)	Increase 5-HT activity		Action on sleep Reported effects on pain	Used in the past. Nefazodone can cause liver problems
Psychostimulants (dextro-amphetamine, methylphenidate, dexmethylphenidate, modafinil)	Increase dopamine activity	Restlessness, agitation, insomnia, nightmares, psychosis, anorexia Arrhythmia, tachycardia hypertension Tolerance, dependence Seizures	Rapid effect Action on pain	Used especially in terminally ill patients

are necessary in specific clinical situations. In fact, cardiovascular adverse effects, seizures, abnormal bleeding, hyponatremia and agranulocytosis should be always taken into consideration as possible serious events in cancer patients [28].

Psychostimulants (e.g. methylphenidate, pemoline, d-amphetamine) have also been used in the treatment of depression in cancer, especially in terminally ill patients, for their rapid onset of action and their effect on attention and concentration problems and on fatigue [29].

Some side effects of ADs may actually be advantageous in cancer patients. For example, if an AD has sedative properties and a patient is having difficulty sleeping, such an agent may be considered for nighttime use (e.g. citalopram). Anxiety is a common symptom in patients with cancer, and ADs with anxiolytic properties may be preferred (e.g. escitalopram, venlafaxine). Patients with appetite problems may benefit from the use of an antidepressant which increases weight (e.g. mirtazapine); patients with psychomotor slowing may benefit from drugs with disinhibiting properties (e.g. bupropion). Patients with neuropathic pain, hot flushes or sexual dysfunction may benefit from specific ADs (see below).

ADs usually start working within two weeks, but there is a great variability in the onset of action in patients with cancer, who may be taking a variety of other medications that impact on antidepressant metabolism, such as steroids, antiemetics and narcotics. Psychostimulants have a shorter latency period, with clinical response in a few days. It is usual that patients are started off on low dosages of ADs to see if there are any side effects such as rash, or adverse drug-drug interactions, before being titrated towards full doses. It may then take more than four–six weeks or even longer for patients to see the full benefit.

Some general guidelines about the use of ADs in people with cancer are summarized in Table 7.2.

Patients with central nervous system involvement (e.g. brain tumours) or with a history of seizures, those with concomitant conditions predisposing to seizures, or those taking other medications that lower seizure threshold are particularly exposed to possible side effects of ADs. Bupropion may induce dose-related seizures and is contraindicated in these patients. Mirtazapine also can lower the threshold for seizures and should be used with caution. There are

Table 7.2   Some guidelines for the use of ADs in cancer patients

- Start the treatment at low doses followed by a period of dose titration to achieve an optimum individualized response (low doses may help to avoid unwanted initial side effects, particularly in patients in poor physical conditions).
- Inform and reassure patients of latency period and possible side effects, in order to avoid premature drop-out, especially if patients are receiving other medications.
- Treat the patient for 4–6 mo in order to avoid relapses or new episodes of depression after remission.
- Regularly monitor the patient's physical variables and concomitant use of medications for cancer (for example, steroids, antiemetics, antibiotics, antiestrogen and chemotherapy agents).
- Discontinue medications by tapering the dose by 50% over a couple of weeks to reduce the risk of withdrawal symptoms that can be distressing and may be mistaken for symptoms of cancer or relapse into depression.
- Reassurance and education of the patients are extremely important in oncology settings.

data to support using citalopram as an antidepressant which does not tend to lower seizure threshold [30].

All TCAs have anticholinergic properties which can cause sedation dry mouth, cardiac arrhythmias, constipation, sexual dysfunction, dizziness, headache, weight gain, and orthostatic hypotension. In patients with significantly dry mucous membranes due to radiation or other treatments, anticholinergic ADs should generally be avoided.

Neutropenia is a rare but possible complication of the use of ADs, including TCAs [31], mianserin [32] and mirtazapine [33], with reported data also for fluoxetine, trazodone, nefazodone and sertraline [34]. Careful examination of numbers of white cells is extremely important in cancer patients receiving chemotherapy, which usually determines neutropenia.

Patients with lung cancer often have dyspnoea, anxiety, pain and, in about 25% of the cases, clinically significant depressive states [35]. Whereas the use of ADs is not generally contraindicated (after careful examination of the possible interactions with other drugs and the physical status of the patient), benzodiazepines should be generally avoided. Although they may provide short-term relief of anxiety, they in fact exacerbate breathing difficulties and, in combination with opioids, may impact quite negatively on pulmonary function.

Patients who have ovarian cancer are particularly susceptible to bowel obstruction. Drugs reducing bowel movements because of their anticholinergic properties, such as TCAs, should be avoided in these patients. ADs should also be carefully evaluated with respect to their action on peristalsis when used in cancer patients receiving opioids for pain.

Cancer patients with compromised liver metabolism or with liver tumours or metastases should be cautiously monitored when receiving ADs, since these drugs are metabolized by the liver. For this reason, liver function tests must be performed at baseline and periodically during therapy. Amongst ADs, nefazodone may cause fatal hepato-toxity and should not be used in patients with liver dysfunction. It also potentially interacts with drugs metabolized by cytochrome P450 isoenzymes.

It is important to avoid anticholinergic medications, such as the TCAs, in patients with delirium. Low-dose antipsychotics (for example, haloperidol, atypical antipsychotics) are often of primary use, while benzodiazepines (apart from delirium tremens or some forms of delirium induced by antibiotics, where they are the key drugs to be used) should be avoided [36].

DRUG INTERACTIONS WITH CHEMOTHERAPY AND ANTICANCER AGENTS

There is still a lack of robust information on the mutual influence between medications used to treat cancer and those used to treat comorbid psychiatric disorders. However, in the last few years some studies have been conducted on this issue and have underlined the need for more attention to this important area [37].

Interferon and Depression

Interferons, a family of proteins that are produced by the immune system, have been shown to have antiproliferative and immuno-modulatory effects, as well as cytotoxic and anti-angiogenic properties. For these reasons, they are used for the treatment of several forms of cancer, such as leukaemia, AIDS-related Kaposi's sarcoma, melanoma, with data also indicating their possible therapeutic effects in renal carcinoma, ovarian cancer and brain tumours [38]. The psychiatric side effects of interferon, especially depression secondary to interferon-alpha, have been known for a long time [39, 40]. Musselman *et al.* [41] explored the efficacy of paroxetine to prevent depression in patients receiving high dose interferon-alpha for malignant melanoma. In a subsequent study, they noticed that depressed mood, anxiety, cognitive dysfunction and pain were more responsive, whereas fatigue and anorexia were less responsive, to paroxetine treatment [42]. Psychostimulants, such as methylphenidate, have also been used to treat depression induced by interferon in cancer patients [43]. Recently, sertraline has been tested not only for its protective role on interferon-induced depression, but also as an adjuvant treatment for melanoma [44].

Tamoxifen and SSRIs

Tamoxifen is a selective oestrogen receptor modulator (SERM) which is used in postmenopausal breast cancer patients who are oestrogen-receptor positive, in order to reduce the risk of recurrence of cancer over time [45]. Tamoxifen, to be clinically active, is converted to 4-hydroxy-tamoxifen (endoxifen) and other active metabolites by cytochrome P450 (CYP) enzymes. More than 80 different major alleles of CYP2D6 gene have been identified, many of which confer decreased or absent CYP2D6 activity, and patients can be divided into poor, intermediate, extensive and ultrarapid metabolizers on the basis of their genotype [46].

Jin *et al.* [47] studied breast cancer patients treated with tamoxifen who were homozygous for a poor metabolizer genotype and had significantly lower serum concentrations of endoxifen than those with active genotype. In retrospective studies evaluating the effect of CYP2D6 genotype on breast cancer outcomes, Goetz *et al.* [48] found that women with oestrogen receptor-positive breast cancer homozygous for the poor metabolizer genotype, treated with tamoxifen monotherapy, were more likely to experience a recurrence of breast cancer than those patients who carried an allele coding for active enzyme. With this as a background and the data showing the role of certain ADs in inhibiting CYPs, Stearns *et al.* [49], in a prospective clinical trial, tested the effects of the co-administration of tamoxifen and paroxetine, often used to treat depression and hot flushes secondary to tamoxifen. The authors found that the use of paroxetine, which inhibits CYP2D6, decreased the plasma concentration of endoxifen, suggesting that CYP2D6 genotype and drug interactions should be considered in all women treated with tamoxifen. Recently, Kelly *et al.* [50] studied 2430 women with breast cancer treated with tamoxifen and a single SSRI. Amongst those who died of breast cancer during follow-up, the authors found that, after adjustment for several potential confounders, absolute increases of 25%, 50%, and 75% in the proportion of time on tamoxifen with overlapping use of paroxetine were associated, respectively, with 24%, 54%, and 91% increases in the risk of death from breast cancer. This confirms that the concomitant use of paroxetine can reduce or suppress the benefit of tamoxifen in women with breast cancer.

In addition to paroxetine, sertraline and venlafaxine have also been involved in reducing the metabolism of tamoxifen [47]. Lash *et al.* [51] indicated no reduction of tamoxifen effectiveness amongst regular citalopram users.

Irinotecan and SSRIs

Irinotecan is a pro-drug that via hydrolysis generates an active compound, SN-38, that works as an inhibitor of topoisomerase I, an important enzyme that cells need in their division process. Irinotecan is used in the treatment of colon cancer [52]. Some data have shown that hypericum (St. John's Wort) can have significant interactions with irinotecan, resulting from the induced expression of the cytochrome

P450 CYP3A4 isoform, with possible deleterious impact on treatment outcome [53]. On the other hand, drugs acting on the serotonergic system (e.g. desipramine, paroxetine and sertraline) are inhibitors of CYP2B6 and may increase the levels/effects of irinotecan. The possible gastrointestinal side effects of SSRIs (e.g. diarrhoea) may aggravate the severe forms of diarrhoea consequent to irinotecan itself. The concomitant use of irinotecan and SSRIs can also have further unexpected side effects, such as rhabdomyolysis, which can be potentially lethal [54].

Serotonin Syndrome

Serotonin syndrome is a potentially life-threatening condition related to ingestion of drugs and drug combinations which alone or synergistically increase serotonin in the body at toxic levels. The symptoms include somatic symptoms (hyperreflexia, myoclonus, tremor), autonomic dysfunction (tachycardia, hypertension, hyperthermia, sweating, shivering, nausea, diarrhoea), cognitive and psychiatric symptoms (agitation, mental confusion, delirium), up to coma [55]. In cancer patients with depression, numerous drugs can produce a serotonin syndrome, including ADs (especially SSRIs and SNRIs), analgesic drugs (e.g. tramadol, opioids) and antiemetics (e.g. 5-HT3 antagonists, such as ondansetron and granisetron). They may act synergically [56, 57], although a clear-cut description of this complication in the oncology setting is lacking.

Steroid Induced Mood Disorders

It is well known that symptoms of hypomania, mania, depression and psychosis may occur during corticosteroid therapy, with symptoms being dose-dependent and generally occurring during the first few weeks of therapy [58–60]. Since corticosteroids are part of cancer treatment, attention should be paid to their possible effects on mood and cognition. Prior psychiatric history and central nervous system complications of cancer should be taken into account [61].

THE USE OF ANTIDEPRESSANTS FOR THE TREATMENT OF OTHER SYMPTOMS IN CANCER PATIENTS

A number of clinical observations and randomized controlled trials have accumulated in the last ten years regarding the role of ADs in the treatment of symptoms and/or dimensions secondary to cancer or cancer therapy that can cause subjective suffering in cancer patients and are often associated with depression. Several data sets are currently available on the use of ADs as adjuvant treatment for pain, hot flushes, pruritus, nausea and vomiting, and fatigue. It shoul be noted, however, that the use of ADs for these symptom dimensions is an 'off label' prescription which is under the responsibility of the physician and must be clearly and fully explained to the patient.

Pain

Pain is one of the most common symptoms and complications in cancer, affecting 30% of all cancer patients, regardless of the stage of the disease, and up to 90% of patients with advanced cancer [62–64]. Pain and depression are closely linked, with a higher risk of mood disorders in patients with uncontrolled pain and an enhanced perception of pain amongst depressed patients [65]. Cancer pain, especially when not properly treated, is accompanied by profound suffering, fear of death without dignity, hopelessness and helplessness, and desire for a hastened death [66]. In several studies, the reciprocal interaction between cancer pain and depression has been repeatedly shown [67], although studies should examine mediating and moderating pathways for this association [68].

ADs have been shown for many years to be effective as adjuvant therapy of chronic pain [69, 70]. There are several reasons explaining the analgesic properties of ADs, including the direct nociceptive effects of serotonin and noradrenaline in the ascending pathways, the enhancement of opioid action, and the enhancement of the inhibitory (analgesic) descending pathways in the medulla [71].

In several psychopharmacological studies examining the efficacy of ADs on depression, pain is one of the most studied outcomes.

Furthermore, both open-label and randomized controlled trials have specifically studied and confirmed the efficacy of ADs in reducing pain (such as bone pain) due to metastases from breast and prostate cancer. TCAs and SNRIs have been the most commonly used [72]. TCAs show analgesic properties at lower doses than those used for treatment of depression, while with SNRIs the efficacy on pain can be obtained with the same doses used to improve mood (venlafaxine, 75–150 mg; duloxetine 60–120 mg).

Hot Flushes

SERM drugs, such as tamoxifen or more recent aromatase inhibitors, administered to breast cancer patients to reduce the risk of cancer recurrence, frequently cause hot flushes, with approximately two thirds of patients experiencing this symptom. Around 60% of patients rate its intensity as severe and 40% as extremely bothersome. Unrelieved hot flushes are related to negative effect, fatigue, sleep difficulties, and overall poor quality of life. This has encouraged the field to develop strategies and guidelines to better manage the problem [73].

ADs, especially SSRIs and SNRIs, have been shown to be effective in treating hot flushes. The first data accumulated regarded the benefit of fluoxetine. In a trial using a double-blind, randomized, two-period (four weeks per period), cross-over methodology to study the efficacy of fluoxetine (20 mg) for treating hot flushes in women with a history of breast cancer or a concern regarding the use of oestrogen (because of breast cancer risk), Loprinzi *et al.* [74] found superiority of the drug over placebo. Controlled trials also indicate that paroxetine [75] and sertraline [76] are superior to placebo in controlling hot flushes in breast cancer patients. However, data concerning the inhibiting effect of paroxetine, sertraline and fluoxetine on the CYP2D6 system in breast cancer patients receiving tamoxifen should induce caution in using these medications for hot flushes.

Likewise, randomized controlled trials using the SNRI venlafaxine showed benefit in ameliorating hot flushes. Women receiving venlafaxine and reporting at least 50% decrease in hot flushes also experienced significant improvement in fatigue, sleep quality, and quality of life [77]. In a randomized controlled trial in breast cancer patients, venlafaxine was shown to be superior to clonidine [78] in reducing hot flushes, but in a further study the medications were equally effective, with more side effects in the venlafaxine arm [79]. Some data indicate that mirtazapine also reduces hot flushes in breast cancer patients [80].

Recent data are accumulating in prostate cancer patients who underwent androgen deprivation [81]. An open-label trial indicated the efficacy of paroxetine in reducing hot flushes in prostate cancer patients [82]. Citalopram has also been shown to be effective in pilot studies [83]. Venlafaxine was also effective in reducing hot flushes in prostate cancer patients, but less effective than cyproterone and medroxyprogesterone [84].

Pruritus

Chronic pruritus of any origin is difficult to treat and has a high impact on patients' quality of life and psychological well-being. During the past years, clinical research has focused on the antipruritic efficacy of centrally acting substances, such as opioid receptor agonists and antagonists as well as on serotonin subtype 3 receptor (5-HT3) antagonists. Mediators of pruritus also include histamine through H1 receptors, and serotonin through 5HT2 and 5HT3 receptors. In some case series and two randomised controlled trials, the SSRIs paroxetine, sertraline and fluoxetine were demonstrated to reduce severe systemic and paraneoplastic pruritus [85, 86]. Also mirtazapine has been shown to reduce pruritus in cancer patients [87, 88].

Nausea and Vomiting/Anorexia

Nausea and vomiting are frequent complications of chemotherapy in cancer patients [89, 90]. Since the early 1970s, drugs with dopaminergic properties have been used to reduce these symptoms in cancer patients. Antipsychotics, especially haloperidol, alone or associated to dexamethazone, are frequently used in reducing nausea and vomiting secondary to chemotherapy [91]. Innovative treatments, especially serotonin antagonists (e.g. ondasetron, granisetron, dolasetron, palonosetron) have been developed to reduce this symptom in oncology

[92]. Recent studies indicated that atypical antipsychotics, in particular olanzapine, are adjuvant drugs for controlling nausea and vomiting secondary to chemotherapy [93].

The concomitant use of AD medications has been recently proven to be useful in the treatment of nausea and vomiting. In open-label studies, e.g. mirtazapine has been shown to improve nausea, sleep disturbance, pain and quality of life, as well as depression in cancer patients [94].

Especially in palliative care patients, anorexia, not necessarily related to nausea, can also be a significant problem related to the advanced phase of cancer. It has been reported that mirtazapine, for its specific effect on appetite, can be helpful for improving this symptom [95].

Fatigue

Fatigue is a symptom affecting 4 to 91% of cancer patients, depending on the specific populations studied and the methods of assessment [96]. A meta-analysis of two studies indicated that methylphenidate was superior to placebo in changing fatigue scores [97]. Placebo-controlled studies of paroxetine indicated a specific benefit on depression but not on cancer-related fatigue [98]. Some open-label studies have found that bupropion, probably because of its activating dopaminergic profile, can also be helpful in cancer-related fatigue [99, 100].

USE OF ANTIDEPRESSANTS AND RISK OF CANCER

At the turn of the century, a debate emerged about a possible association of chronic use of ADs, especially TCAs and SSRIs, with an increased risk of cancer, in particular breast cancer [101–103]. More recent epidemiological data have not confirmed this association [104–106]. In a recent study conducted in Finland, no clear evidence of either positive or negative association between usage of ADs and cancer could be found [107]. From the opposite perspective, there have been recent reports that ADs, particularly SSRIs and possibly TCAs, may be associated with a reduced risk of cancer. Starting from preliminary studies on the use of fluoxetine and citalopram [108], SSRIs have been found to inhibit colorectal tumour cells that are dependent on serotonin for their growth, through an antipromoter action or direct cytotoxic effect. In multi-drug resistant cases of human colon cancer, *in vitro* fluoxetine enhanced by 10-fold the cytotoxicity activity of the chemotherapeutic agent doxorubicin, increasing its intracellular accumulation and decreasing its efflux [109]. *In vivo*, combination treatment with doxorubicin and fluoxetine significantly slowed-down tumour progression (vs. doxorubicin alone) [110, 111].

CONCLUSIONS

Depressive disorders in cancer patients represent a significant clinical problem, whether a categorical (e.g. ICD-10, DSM-IV) or a dimensional (e.g. Diagnostic Criteria for Psychosomatic Research) approach is used [112, 113]. The prevalence is high in all phases of illness and the consequences are severe for both the patient and the family.

In spite of the limitations of currently available randomized controlled trials, including small sample sizes, high withdrawal rates and infrequent use of structured diagnostic interviews [25], the efficacy of ADs in depressed patients with cancer can be considered well documented, and their tolerability seems to be good, particularly with new drugs [114]. The evidence of some adverse effects should be interpreted in the light of the multiple treatments that cancer patients usually receive. Furthermore, ADs have been shown to be helpful in treating not only depression but several other symptoms which are common in cancer patients, especially pain and hot flushes.

Further research evidence is needed on the efficacy, effectiveness and safety of ADs in the different settings of oncology (inpatient units, outpatient clinics and palliative care units) and types of cancer. In fact, cancer is a very heterogeneous disease, with different genetic, endocrinological and immunological concomitants. Finally, more information is needed about the interactions between ADs and the variety of drugs, especially chemotherapeutic agents, cancer patients receive.

REFERENCES

1. McDaniel, J.S., Musselman, D.L., Porter, M.R. *et al.* (1995) Depression in patients with cancer. Diagnosis, biology, and treatment. *Arch. Gen. Psychiatry*, **52**, 89–99.
2. Chochinov, H.M. (2001) Depression in cancer patients. *Lancet Oncol.*, **2**, 499–505.
3. Massie, M.J. (2004) Prevalence of depression in patients with cancer. *J. Natl. Cancer Inst. Monogr.*, **32**, 57–71.
4. Grassi, L., Holland, J.C., Johansen, C. *et al.* (2005) Psychiatric concomitants of cancer, screening procedures, and training of health care professionals in oncology: the paradigms of psycho-oncology in the psychiatry field, in *Advances in Psychiatry*, vol. 2 (ed. G.N. Christodoulou), Beta Publishing, Athens, pp. 59–66.
5. Greenberg, D.B. (2004) Barriers to the treatment of depression in cancer patients. *J. Natl. Cancer Inst. Monogr.*, **32**, 127–135.
6. Spoletini, I., Gianni, W., Repetto, L. *et al.* (2008) Depression and cancer: an unexplored and unresolved emergent issue in elderly patients. *Crit. Rev. Oncol. Hematol.*, **65**, 143–155.
7. Newport, D.J. and Nemeroff, C.B. (1998) Assessment and treatment of depression in the cancer patient. *J. Psychosom. Res.*, **45**, 215–237.
8. National Comprehensive Cancer Network. Distress management. www.nccn.org.
9. Bultz, B.D. and Carlson, L.E. (2006) Emotional distress: the sixth vital sign – future directions in cancer care. *Psychooncology*, **15**, 93–95.
10. Sharpe, M., Strong, V., Allen, K. *et al.* (2004) Major depression in outpatients attending a regional cancer centre: screening and unmet treatment needs. *Br. J. Cancer*, **90**, 314–320.
11. Sharpe, M., Strong, V., Allen, K. *et al.* (2004) Management of major depression in outpatients attending a cancer centre: a preliminary evaluation of a multicomponent cancer nurse-delivered intervention. *Br. J. Cancer*, **90**, 310–313.
12. Strong, V., Waters, R., Hibberd, C. *et al.* (2008) Management of depression for people with cancer (SMaRT oncology 1): a randomised trial. *Lancet*, **372**, 40–48.
13. Shimizu, K., Ishibashi, Y., Umezawa, S., *et al.* Feasibility and usefulness of the 'Distress Screening Program in Ambulatory Care' in clinical oncology practice. *Psychooncology* (in press).
14. Grassi, L. and Riba, M. (2009) New frontiers and challenges of psychiatry in oncology and palliative care, in *Advances in Psychiatry*,

vol. 3 (eds G.N. Christodoulou, M. Jorge and J.E. Mezzich), Beta Publishers, Athens, pp. 105–114.

15. Shimizu, K., Akechi, T., Shimamoto, M. *et al.* (2007) Can psychiatric intervention improve major depression in very near end-of-life cancer patients? *Palliat. Support Care*, **5**, 3–9.

16. Jaeger, H., Morrow, G.R., Carpenter, P.J. and Brescia, F. (1985) A survey of psychotropic drug utilization by patients with advanced neoplastic disease. *Gen. Hosp. Psychiatry*, **7**, 353–360.

17. Peterson, L.G., Leipman, M. and Bongar, B. (1987) Psychotropic medications in patients with cancer. *Gen. Hosp. Psychiatry*, **9**, 313–323.

18. Stiefel, F.C., Kornblith, A.B. and Holland, J.C. (1990) Changes in prescription patterns of psychotropic drugs for cancer patients during a 10-year period. *Cancer*, **65**, 1048–1053.

19. Ashbury, F.D., Madlensky, L., Raich, P. *et al.* (2003) Antidepressant prescribing in community cancer care. *Support. Care Cancer*, **11**, 278–285.

20. Coyne, J.C., Palmer, S.C., Shapiro, P.J. *et al.* (2004) Distress, psychiatric morbidity, and prescriptions for psychotropic medication in a breast cancer waiting room sample. *Gen. Hosp. Psychiatry*, **26**, 121–128.

21. Hewitt, M. and Rowland, J.H. (2002) Mental health service use among adult cancer survivors: analyses of the National Health Interview Survey. *J. Clin. Oncol.*, **20**, 4581–4590.

22. Kadan-Lottick, N.S., Vanderwerker, L.C., Block, S.D. *et al.* (2005) Psychiatric disorders and mental health service use in patients with advanced cancer: a report from the Coping with Cancer Study. *Cancer*, **104**, 2872–2881.

23. Okamura, M., Akizuki, N., Nakano, T. *et al.* (2008) Clinical experience of the use of a pharmacological treatment algorithm for major depressive disorder in patients with advanced cancer. *Psychooncology*, **17**, 154–160.

24. Rayner, L., Higginson, I.J., Price, A. and Hotopf, M. (2009) The management of depression in palliative care: draft European clinical guidelines. EPCRC Depression Guideline Expert Group, London.

25. Rodin, G., Lloyd, N., Katz, M. *et al.* (2007) The treatment of depression in cancer patients: a systematic review. *Support. Care Cancer*, **15**, 123–136.

26. Berney, A., Stiefel, F., Mazzocato, C. and Buclin, T. (1999) Psychopharmacology in supportive care in cancer: a review for the clinician. III. Antidepressants. *Support. Care Cancer*, **7**, 379–385.

27. Pirl, W.F. (2004) Evidence report on the occurrence, assessment, and treatment of depression in cancer patients. *J. Natl. Cancer Inst. Monogr.*, **32**, 32–39.

28. Mago, R., Mahajan, R. and Thase, M.E. (2008) Medically serious adverse effects of newer antidepressants. *Curr. Psychiatry Rep.*, **10**, 249–257.

29. Homsi, J., Walsh, D. and Nelson, K.A. (2000) Psychostimulants in supportive care. *Support. Care Cancer*, **8**, 385–397.

30. Lazure, K.E., Lydiatt, W.M., Denman, D. and Burke, W.J. (2009) Association between depression and survival or disease recurrence in patients with head and neck cancer enrolled in a depression prevention trial. *Head Neck*, **31**, 888–892.

31. Albertini, R.S. and Penders, T.M. (1978) Agranulocytosis associated with tricyclics. *J. Clin. Psychiatry*, **39**, 483–485.

32. Adams, P.C., Robinson, A., Reid, M.M. *et al.* (1983) Blood dyscrasias and mianserin. *Postgrad. Med. J.*, **59**, 31–33.

33. Kasper, S., Praschak-Rieder, N., Tauscher, J. and Wolf, R. (1997) A risk-benefit assessment of mirtazapine in the treatment of depression. *Drug Saf.*, **17**, 251–264.

34. Duggal, H.S. and Singh, I. (2005) Psychotropic drug-induced neutropenia. *Drugs Today*, **41**, 517–526.

35. Steinberg, T., Roseman, M., Kasymjanova, G. *et al.* (2009) Prevalence of emotional distress in newly diagnosed lung cancer patients. *Support. Care Cancer*, **17**, 1493–1497.

36. Caraceni, A. and Grassi, L. (2003) *Delirium: Acute Confusional States in Palliative Medicine*, Oxford University Press, Oxford.

37. Yap, K.Y., Tay, W.L., Chui, W.K. and Chan, A., Clinically relevant drug interactions between anticancer drugs and psychotropic agents. *Eur. J. Cancer Care* (in press).

38. Bracarda, S., Eggermont, A.M. and Samuelsson, J., Redefining the role of interferon in the treatment of malignant diseases. *Eur. J. Cancer*, **46**, 284–97.

39. Valentine, A.D. and Meyers, C.A. (2005) Neurobehavioral effects of interferon therapy. *Curr. Psychiatry Rep.*, **7**, 391–395.

40. Patten, S.B. (2006) Psychiatric side effects of interferon treatment. *Curr. Drug Saf.*, **1**, 143–150.

41. Musselman, D.L., Lawson, D.H., Gumnick, J.F. *et al.* (2001) Paroxetine for the prevention of depression induced by high-dose interferon alfa. *N. Engl. J. Med.*, **344**, 961–966.

42. Capuron, L., Gumnick, J.F., Musselman, D.L. *et al.* (2002) Neurobehavioral effects of interferon-alpha in cancer patients: phenomenology

and paroxetine responsiveness of symptom dimensions. *Neuropsychopharmacology*, **26**, 643–652.

43. Camacho, A. and Ng, B. (2006) Methylphenidate for alpha-interferon induced depression. *J. Psychopharmacol.*, **20**, 687–689.

44. Reddy, K.K., Lefkove, B., Chen, L.B. *et al.* (2008) The antidepressant sertraline downregulates Akt and has activity against melanoma cells. *Pigment Cell Melanoma Res.*, **21**, 451–456.

45. Nelson, H.D., Fu, R., Griffin, J.C. *et al.* (2009) Systematic review: comparative effectiveness of medications to reduce risk for primary breast cancer. *Ann. Intern. Med.*, **151**, 703–715.

46. Henry, N.L., Stearns, V., Flockhart, D.A. *et al.* (2008) Drug interactions and pharmacogenomics in the treatment of breast cancer and depression. *Am. J. Psychiatry*, **165**, 1251–1255.

47. Jin, Y., Desta, Z., Stearns, V. *et al.* (2005) CYP2D6 genotype, antidepressant use, and tamoxifen metabolism during adjuvant breast cancer treatment. *J. Natl. Cancer Inst.*, **97** 30–39.

48. Goetz, M.P., Rae, J.M., Suman, V.J. *et al.* (2005) Pharmacogenetics of tamoxifen biotransformation is associated with clinical outcomes of efficacy and hot flushes. *J. Clin. Oncol.*, **23**, 9312–9318.

49. Stearns, V., Johnson, M.D., Rae, J.M. *et al.* (2003) Active tamoxifen metabolite plasma concentrations after coadministration of tamoxifen and the selective serotonin reuptake inhibitor paroxetine. *J. Natl. Cancer Inst.*, **95**, 1758–1764.

50. Kelly, C.M., Juurlink, D.N., Gomes, T., *et al.* Selective serotonin reuptake inhibitors and breast cancer mortality in women receiving tamoxifen: a population based cohort study. *BMJ* (in press).

51. Lash, T.L., Pedersen, L., Cronin-Fenton, D. *et al.* (2008) Tamoxifen's protection against breast cancer recurrence is not reduced by concurrent use of the SSRI citalopram. *Br. J. Cancer*, **99**, 616–621.

52. Weekes, J., Lam, A.K., Sebesan, S. and Ho, Y.H. (2009) Irinotecan therapy and molecular targets in colorectal cancer: a systemic review. *World J. Gastroenterol.*, **15**, 3597–3602.

53. Mathijssen, R.H., Verweij, J., de Bruijn, P. *et al.* (2002) Effects of St. John's Wort on irinotecan metabolism. *J. Natl. Cancer Inst.*, **94**, 1247–1249.

54. Richards, S., Umbreit, J.N., Fanucchi, M.P. *et al.* (2003) Selective serotonin reuptake inhibitor-induced rhabdomyolysis associated with irinotecan. *South Med. J.*, **96**, 1031–1033.

55. Kim, H.F. and Fisch, M.J. (2006) Antidepressant use in ambulatory cancer patients. *Curr. Oncol. Rep.*, **8**, 275–281.

56. Lee, J., Franz, L. and Goforth, H.W. (2009) Serotonin syndrome in a chronic-pain patient receiving concurrent methadone, ciprofloxacin, and venlafaxine. *Psychosomatics*, **50**, 638–639.

57. Takeshita, J. and Litzinger, M.H. (2009) Serotonin syndrome associated with tramadol. *Prim. Care Companion J. Clin. Psychiatry*, **11**, 273.

58. Brown, E.S. and Suppes, T. (1998) Mood symptoms during corticosteroid therapy: a review. *Harv. Rev. Psychiatry*, **5**, 239–246.

59. Brown, E.S. and Chandler, P.A. (2001) Mood and cognitive changes during systemic corticosteroid therapy. *Prim. Care Companion J. Clin. Psychiatry*, **3**, 17–21.

60. Wada, K., Yamada, N., Sato, T. *et al.* (2001) Corticosteroid-induced psychotic and mood disorders: diagnosis defined by DSM-IV and clinical pictures. *Psychosomatics*, **42**, 461–466.

61. Stiefel, F.C., Breitbart, W.S. and Holland, J.C. (1989) Corticosteroids in cancer: neuropsychiatric complications. *Cancer Invest.*, **7**, 479–491.

62. Goudas, L.C., Bloch, R., Gialeli-Goudas, M. *et al.* (2005) The epidemiology of cancer pain. *Cancer Invest.*, **23**, 182–190.

63. van den Beuken-van Everdingen, M.H., de Rijke, J.M., Kessels, A.G. *et al.* (2007) Prevalence of pain in patients with cancer: a systematic review of the past 40 years. *Ann. Oncol.*, **18**, 1437–1449.

64. Breivik, H., Cherny, N., Collett, B. *et al.* (2009) Cancer-related pain: a pan-European survey of prevalence, treatment, and patient attitudes. *Ann. Oncol.*, **20**, 1420–1433.

65. Bair, M.J., Robinson, R.L., Katon, W. and Kroenke, K. (2003) Depression and pain comorbidity: a literature review. *Arch. Intern. Med.*, **163**, 2433–2445.

66. Breitbart, W., Payne, D. and Passik, S. (2004) Psychological and psychiatric interventions in pain control, in *Oxford Textbook of Palliative Medicine*, 3rd edn (eds. D. Doyle, G. Hanks, N. Cherny and K. Calman), Oxford University Press, New York, pp. 424–438.

67. Gagliese, L., Gauthier, L.R. and Rodin, G. (2007) Cancer pain and depression: a systematic review of age-related patterns. *Pain Res. Manag.*, **12**, 205–211.

68. Laird, B.J., Boyd, A.C., Colvin, L.A. and Fallon, M.T. (2009) Are cancer pain and depression interdependent? A systematic review. *Psychooncology*, **18**, 459–464.

69. Barkin, R.L. and Fawcett, J. (2000) The management challenges of chronic pain: the role of antidepressants. *Am. J. Ther.*, **7**, 31–47.

70. Kroenke, K., Krebs, E.E. and Bair, M.J. (2009) Pharmacotherapy of chronic pain: a synthesis of recommendations from systematic reviews. *Gen. Hosp. Psychiatry*, **31**, 206–219.

71. Blier, P. and Abbott, F.V. (2001) Putative mechanisms of action of antidepressant drugs in affective and anxiety disorders and pain. *J. Psychiatry Neurosci.*, **26**, 37–43.

72. Lussier, D., Huskey, A.G. and Portenoy, R.K. (2004) Adjuvant analgesics in cancer pain management. *Oncologist*, **9**, 571–591.

73. Hickey, M., Saunders, C., Partridge, A. *et al.* (2008) Practical clinical guidelines for assessing and managing menopausal symptoms after breast cancer. *Ann. Oncol.*, **19**, 1669–1680.

74. Loprinzi, C.L., Sloan, J.A., Perez, E.A. *et al.* (2002) Phase III evaluation of fluoxetine for treatment of hot flushes. *J. Clin. Oncol.*, **20**, 1578–1583.

75. Stearns, V., Slack, R., Greep, N. *et al.* (2005) Paroxetine is an effective treatment for hot flushes: results from a prospective randomized clinical trial. *J. Clin. Oncol.*, **23**, 6919–6930.

76. Kimmick, G.G., Lovato, J., McQuellon, R. *et al.* (2006) Randomized, double-blind, placebo-controlled, crossover study of sertraline (Zoloft) for the treatment of hot flushes in women with early stage breast cancer taking tamoxifen. *Breast J.*, **12**, 114–122.

77. Carpenter, J.S., Storniolo, A.M., Johns, S. *et al.* (2007) Randomized, double-blind, placebo-controlled crossover trials of venlafaxine for hot flushes after breast cancer. *Oncologist*, **12**, 124–135.

78. Loibl, S., Schwedler, K., von Minckwitz, G. *et al.* (2007) Venlafaxine is superior to clonidine as treatment of hot flushes in breast cancer patients—a double-blind, randomized study. *Ann. Oncol.*, **18**, 689–693.

79. Buijs, C., Mom, C.H., Willemse, P.H. *et al.* (2009) Venlafaxine versus clonidine for the treatment of hot flushes in breast cancer patients: a double-blind, randomized cross-over study. *Breast Cancer Res. Treat.*, **115**, 573–580.

80. Biglia, N., Kubatzki, F., Sgandurra, P. *et al.* (2007) Mirtazapine for the treatment of hot flushes in breast cancer survivors: a prospective pilot trial. *Breast J.*, **13**, 490–495.

81. Stearns, V. (2004) Management of hot flushes in breast cancer survivors and men with prostate cancer. *Curr. Oncol. Rep.*, **6**, 285–290.

82. Naoe, M., Ogawa, Y., Shichijo, T. *et al.* (2006) Pilot evaluation of selective serotonin reuptake inhibitor antidepressants in hot flush patients under androgen-deprivation therapy for prostate cancer. *Prostate Cancer Prostatic Dis.*, **9**, 275–278.

83. Barton, D.L., Loprinzi, C.L., Novotny, P. *et al.* (2003) Pilot evaluation of citalopram for the relief of hot flushes. *J. Support Oncol.*, **1**, 47–51.

84. Irani, J., Salomon, L., Oba, R., *et al.* Efficacy of venlafaxine, medroxyprogesterone acetate, and cyproterone acetate for the treatment of

vasomotor hot flushes in men taking gonadotropin-releasing hormone analogues for prostate cancer: a double-blind, randomised trial. *Lancet Oncol.* **11**, 147–54.

85. Zylicz, Z., Smits, C. and Krajnik, M. (1998) Paroxetine for pruritus in advanced cancer. *J. Pain Symptom Manag.*, **16**, 121–124.

86. Zylicz, Z., Krajnik, M., Sorge, A.A. and Costantini, M. (2003) Paroxetine in the treatment of severe non-dermatological pruritus: a randomized, controlled trial. *J. Pain Symptom Manag.*, **26**, 1105–1112.

87. Davis, M.P., Frandsen, J.L., Walsh, D. *et al.* (2003) Mirtazapine for pruritus. *J. Pain Symptom Manag.*, **25**, 288–291.

88. Demierre, M.F. and Taverna, J. (2006) Mirtazapine and gabapentin for reducing pruritus in cutaneous T-cell lymphoma. *J. Am. Acad. Dermatol.*, **55**, 543–544.

89. Schwartzberg, L. (2006) Chemotherapy-induced nausea and vomiting: state of the art in 2006. *J. Support Oncol.*, **4** (Suppl. 1), 3–8.

90. Lohr, L. (2008) Chemotherapy-induced nausea and vomiting. *Cancer J.*, **14**, 85–93.

91. Critchley, P., Plach, N., Grantham, M. *et al.* (2001) Efficacy of haloperidol in the treatment of nausea and vomiting in the palliative patient: a systematic review. *J. Pain Symptom Manag.*, **22**, 631–634.

92. Navari, R.M. (2009) Pharmacological management of chemotherapy-induced nausea and vomiting: focus on recent developments. *Drugs*, **69**, 515–533.

93. Tan, L., Liu, J., Liu, X. *et al.* (2009) Clinical research of olanzapine for prevention of chemotherapy-induced nausea and vomiting. *J. Exp. Clin. Cancer Res.*, **28**, 131.

94. Kim, S.W., Shin, I.S., Kim, J.M. *et al.* (2008) Effectiveness of mirtazapine for nausea and insomnia in cancer patients with depression. *Psychiatry Clin. Neurosci.*, **62**, 75–83.

95. Riechelmann, R.P., Burman, D., Tannock, I.F., *et al.* Phase II trial of mirtazapine for cancer-related cachexia and anorexia. *Am. J. Hosp. Palliat. Care* (in press).

96. Breitbart, W. and Alici-Evcimen, Y. (2007) Update on psychotropic medications for cancer-related fatigue. *J. Natl. Compr. Canc. Netw.*, **5**, 1081–1091.

97. Minton, O., Richardson, A., Sharpe, M. *et al.* (2008) A systematic review and meta-analysis of the pharmacological treatment of cancer-related fatigue. *J. Natl. Cancer Inst.*, **100**, 1155–1166.

98. Morrow, G.R., Hickok, J.T., Roscoe, J.A. *et al.* (2003) Differential effects of paroxetine on fatigue and depression: a randomized, double-

blind trial from the University of Rochester Cancer Center Community Clinical Oncology Program. *J. Clin. Oncol.*, **21**, 4635–4641.

99. Moss, E.L., Simpson, J.S., Pelletier, G. and Forsyth, P. (2006) An open-label study of the effects of bupropion SR on fatigue, depression and quality of life of mixed-site cancer patients and their partners. *Psychooncology*, **15**, 259–267.

100. Cullum, J.L., Wojciechowski, A.E., Pelletier, G. and Simpson, J.S. (2004) Bupropion sustained release treatment reduces fatigue in cancer patients. *Can. J. Psychiatry*, **49** (2), 139–144.

101. Kelly, J.P., Rosenberg, L., Palmer, J.R. *et al.* (1999) Risk of breast cancer according to use of antidepressants, phenothiazines, and anti-histamines. *Am. J. Epidemiol.*, **150**, 861–868.

102. Cotterchio, M., Kreiger, N., Darlington, G. and Steingart, A. (2000) Antidepressant medication use and breast cancer risk. *Am. J. Epidemiol.*, **151**, 951–957.

103. Bahl, S., Cotterchio, M. and Kreiger, N. (2003) Use of antidepressant medications and the possible association with breast cancer risk. A review. *Psychother. Psychosom.*, **72**, 185–194.

104. Wang, P.S., Walker, A.M., Tsuang, M.T. *et al.* (2001) Antidepressant use and the risk of breast cancer: a non-association. *J. Clin. Epidemiol.*, **54**, 728–734.

105. Lawlor, D.A., Jüni, P., Ebrahim, S. and Egger, M. (2003) Systematic review of the epidemiologic and trial evidence of an association between antidepressant medication and breast cancer. *J. Clin. Epidemiol.*, **56**, 155–163.

106. Wernli, K.J., Hampton, J.M., Trentham-Dietz, A. and Newcomb, P.A. (2009) Antidepressant medication use and breast cancer risk. *Pharmacoepidemiol. Drug Saf.*, **18**, 284–290.

107. Haukka, J., Sankila, R., Klaukka, T. *et al.* (2009) Incidence of cancer and antidepressant medication: record linkage study. *Int. J. Cancer*, **126**, 285–296.

108. Tutton, P.J. and Barkla, D.H. (1982) Influence of inhibitors of serotonin uptake on intestinal epithelium and colorectal carcinomas. *Br. J. Cancer*, **46**, 260–265.

109. Argov, M., Kashi, R., Peer, D. and Margalit, R. (2009) Treatment of resistant human colon cancer xenografts by a fluoxetine-doxorubicin combination enhances therapeutic responses comparable to an aggressive bevacizumab regimen. *Cancer Lett.*, **274**, 118–125.

110. Xu, W., Tamim, H., Shapiro, S. *et al.* (2006) Use of antidepressants and risk of colorectal cancer: a nested case-control study. *Lancet Oncol.*, **7**, 301–308.

111. Coogan, P.F., Strom, B.L. and Rosenberg, L. (2009) Antidepressant use and colorectal cancer risk. *Pharmacoepidemiol Drug Saf.*, **18**, 1111–1114.

112. Fabbri, S., Fava, G.A., Sirri, L. and Wise, T.N. (2007) Development of a new assessment strategy in psychosomatic medicine: the Diagnostic Criteria for Psychosomatic Research, in *Psychological Factors Affecting Medical Conditions. A New Classification for DSM-V* (eds. P. Porcelli and N. Sonino), Karger, Basel, pp. 1–20.

113. Grassi, L., Biancosino, B., Marmai, L. *et al.* (2007) Psychological factors affecting oncology conditions, in *Psychological Factors Affecting Medical Conditions. A New Classification for DSM-V* (eds. P. Porcelli and N. Sonino), Karger, Basel, pp. 57–71.

114. Williams, S. and Dale, J. (2006) The effectiveness of treatment for depression/depressive symptoms in adults with cancer: a systematic review. *Br. J. Cancer*, **94**, 372–390.

CHAPTER 8

Psychotherapy for Depression in Cancer and Palliative Care

David W. Kissane and Tomer Levin

*Department of Psychiatry and Behavioral Sciences,
Memorial Sloan-Kettering Cancer Center, New York, NY, USA*

Sarah Hales, Christopher Lo and Gary Rodin

*Department of Psychosocial Oncology and Palliative Care,
Princess Margaret Hospital, Toronto, ON, Canada*

Evidence-based medicine advocates the use of effective interventions ahead of treatments not shown to have been efficacious. Jacobsen and Jim suggest that psychosocial cancer care that is ineffective is worse than no care at all [1]. This highlights the importance of assessing an intervention's impact rather than relying on good intentions alone.

This chapter focuses on evidence-based psychotherapies, which have the largest probability of reproducible efficacy. We begin with individually-focused therapies for patients with early stage cancer, move to systemic therapies (couple, group and family) that bridge across all stages of cancer and conclude with psychotherapy for advanced cancer, including patients receiving palliative care.

Depression and Cancer   Edited by David W. Kissane, Mario Maj and Norman Sartorius
© 2011 John Wiley & Sons, Ltd

PSYCHOTHERAPIES IN EARLY STAGE CANCER

Individually-Focused Psychotherapies

Issues and Symptoms

Before implementing a psychotherapeutic strategy, it is important to develop a comprehensive formulation of the case and consider the differential diagnosis, as the depression phenotype in cancer is heterogeneous. In other words, depressive symptoms must be understood in the context of the whole person, the cancer narrative and the biology of the illness. To illustrate, consider a person meeting typical DSM-IV criteria for major depression (decreased mood, anhedonia, loss of appetite, sleep disturbances, psychomotor slowing or agitation, decreased energy, guilt, decreased concentration and suicidal ideation [2]). The psychotherapeutic approach will vary if the depressive symptoms occur against a backdrop of treatment with prednisone (associated with mood disorders), poorly managed pain, relationship difficulties, childhood sexual abuse, an axis II diagnosis, chronic dysthymia, postnatal depression, a family history of bipolar disorder and so forth. Thus, depression must be viewed within the biopsychosocial context of the person, rather than as an isolated symptom cluster.

The differential diagnosis for major depression in a person with cancer includes mood disorder due to a medical condition, substance-induced mood disorder, dementia, delirium and bipolar disorder. In these cases, the primary treatment may not necessarily be psychotherapy, but rather treatment of the underlying condition. The category of mood disorder due to a medical condition may be problematic in some respects. Although it requires a temporal association between the onset and course of the medical condition and depression, psychiatric symptoms of a medical illness may antedate its clinical recognition. Additionally, since depression is most often multi-determined, correction of the medical illness may not eliminate the depressive symptoms. Similarly, depression may predate substance-induced mood disorder, and treatment of the substance abuse does not necessarily resolve the depressive symptoms, which may require specific psychotherapeutic treatment. Comorbid substance abuse may also benefit from specific drug treatments, inpatient detoxification or psychotherapies, such as motivational interviewing, which have been shown to be efficacious in this subgroup [3].

Cognitive Therapy

Cognitive therapy (CT) or cognitive-behavioural therapy (CBT) is based on the cognitive hypothesis that it is not a particular situation that causes an emotional reaction but rather how a person perceives that situation [4]. For example, one person who undergoes diagnostic imaging for a likely malignancy may feel depressed because he worries that he will be dependent on his family. Another person in the same situation may feel relief and think 'at last we will find out the reason for this pain and work out a way to treat it'. Thus, a triggering situation leads to an 'automatic thought', which then generates a response that can be emotional (e.g. worry), behavioural (e.g. withdrawal) or physiological (e.g. gastrointestinal discomfort). Reframing of dysfunctional automatic thoughts is an important component of CT's therapeutic work. These maladaptive cancer-related cognitions can be characterized by an absolute or over-generalized quality, reflected in a statement such as '*Everything* reminds me of the cancer'. The therapist's aim is to moderate the intensity of such cognitive thinking biases by engaging the patient in a consideration of more reasonable alternatives. Table 8.1 illustrates some realistic reframes.

Central to CT is the cognitive formulation, which is often laid out in a tabular format known as a Dysfunctional Thought Record [5]. This assists the clinician in defining potential treatment goals, which are negotiated collaboratively using measurable outcomes [6]. Some examples of depression treatment goals are a 50% reduction in depression severity measured on a scale such as the Patient Health Questionnaire (PHQ-9) [7], improvement in communication with spouse (where relationship conflict is a trigger for depression) and behavioural activation goals such as returning to work or resuming social activities (e.g. singing in the choir).

Empiricism is a central stance of CT. For example, the therapist might propose the hypothesis that relationship conflict is worsening

Table 8.1 Cognitive therapy examples of realistic reframes used to counter the negative thinking met in cancer care

Nature of the cognitive distortion	Realistic response upon reframing
Catastrophization: 'The cancer is certain to return. My situation is hopeless. I might as well give up'.	'My oncologist gives me a good prognosis. I'm fortunate my cancer has been curable'.
Magnification: 'This back pain will be the cancer back again. I'm in trouble'.	'I've been gardening. The backache will likely be gone tomorrow. I'll tell my doctor if it persists next week'.
All-or-nothing thinking: 'If I can't be cured, there is no point in doing anything'.	'Although my cancer is incurable, it can be contained by treatment for several years'.
Selective attention: 'I fear the side effects of chemotherapy will make me miserable'.	'Chemotherapy reduces the risk of recurrence considerably. It is worth the burden of side effects to gain this benefit'.
Pessimism, predicting the future: 'I'm sure to lose my hair and then my partner will leave me'.	'*Look good, feel better* teaches me confidence in wearing a wig. I'll have fun with my husband exploring new styles'.
Use of verbs 'should' and 'ought': 'I should be able to do everything I did before cancer. I ought to cope better than this'.	'Chemotherapy causes a mild anaemia with resultant fatigue. Gentle exercise will protect against muscle wasting'.
Labelling: 'I'm pathetic. I'm so spineless'.	'Actually, this radiation causes a lot of inflammation. It makes sense to use the painkillers prescribed. I'll get there'.
Personalization: 'It's not surprising I got cancer. It must be my fault'.	'Random DNA changes cause cancer. It affects every family. It is an old myth that stress causes cancer'.
Illogical thinking: 'If I don't feel happier soon, I'll never get better from this cancer'.	'Antidepressants take a few days to begin working. I need patience for the medication to help'.
Emotional reasoning: 'Because I feel inadequate, I must be doing a poor job at work during this chemotherapy treatment'.	'I'm working on boosting my self-esteem. However, it is not connected to how others see me. My colleagues at work are supportive'.

the depression symptoms. Evidence for and against this hypothesis is analysed with the patient and strategies to improve the relationship are implemented. Data is collected to measure the success of the strategies and, therefore, to either support or refute the hypothesis. Another benefit of CT in psycho-oncology is that it promotes autonomy and self-management, which is often a desirable outcome in helping patients to cope better with chronic illnesses [8]. Generally, it takes about 12 sessions to treat uncomplicated major depression, although a degree of symptom relief is often achieved after four sessions. Sessions may be weekly at first and then, once symptom relief is achieved, consolidation or maintenance therapy may consist of regular but less frequent sessions, such as on a monthly basis, or booster sessions which are arranged when depressive symptoms recur or when newer problems emerge.

Evidence supporting the efficacy of CBT for depression can be found in meta-analyses of multiple randomized controlled trials in cancer survivors [9, 10]. A newer paradigm involves the use of a psychotherapy intervention to prevent depressive outcomes in cancer patients at high risk for depression, based on a prior history of depression or anxiety. Pitceathly *et al.* [11] demonstrated that a short CBT intervention (three sessions), administered by trained nurses, significantly reduced the rate of depression in patients who were at high risk, but not depressed at baseline. The first session lasting 90 minutes was conducted face to face, but subsequent sessions were conducted by phone. Significant effects were noted up to six months after the intervention. The demonstration of the efficacy of well-trained nurse therapists is another welcome advancement that will allow more patients access to depression treatment.

Problem-Solving Therapy

This therapy was distilled from overarching CBT principles and is based on the hypothesis that more efficient problem solving or improved coping results in less psychological distress. The standard 90 minutes × 10 sessions programme teaches patients to define the problem, brainstorm possible options, evaluate potential solutions, implement solutions, monitor their degree of success, and fine-tune them. A family member can be conscripted as a coach, which is logical, as most people solve problems collaboratively and cancer affects the whole family. Problem-solving attitudes are examined. To illustrate, a person may believe that *all* of his problems are due to the cancer (which is challenged by the view that the cancer cannot be blamed for every single problem) or that *no one* can help (while, in fact, many patients are helped) [12]. In a randomized controlled study, problem solving was effective in reducing depressive symptoms ($p < 0.05$) versus a waiting list control, a benefit that was still robust at one year [13].

Psychoeducational Interventions

Psychoeducational interventions provide verbal, written or visual information to help patients orientate themselves to novel oncology situations. Acquisition of new knowledge is essential to help patients navigate unfamiliar medical systems and new treatment processes, which can be quite overwhelming. For example, one psychoeducation study involved an orientation tour of the clinic, written resources for coping (e.g. support groups) and a question and answer meeting with a therapist. Devine and Westlake's meta-analysis of 116 psychoeducational studies [14] reported a moderate effect size ($d = 0.54$, 95% $CI = 0.43–0.65$) for amelioration of depression, and a systematic qualitative analysis [15] found positive results in 63% of studies reviewed. A related concept is that of patient navigators, a barrier-focused intervention that helps patients complete a discrete episode of cancer-related care [16]. It contains elements that overlap with psychoeducation, all of which point to the fact that better orientation and support in unfamiliar medical situations can help shape expectations and reduce demoralization and helplessness.

Relaxation Therapies

Relaxation interventions are amongst the most widely used psycho-social services offered to cancer patients and are particularly useful for managing 'here and now' behaviours or distress associated with cancer treatments. Luebbert's meta-analysis [17] estimated a moderate effect size of relaxation on depression (d = 0.54, 95% CI = 0.30–0.78). Jacobsen *et al.* [18] developed a stress management intervention for chemotherapy patients that was self-administered, using print and audio instructions. Using three techniques (paced abdominal breathing, progressive muscle relaxation with guided imagery and coping self-statements), depression and anxiety symptoms were significantly less than in the control group after two, three and four cycles of chemotherapy.

Behavioural Activation

Behavioural activation (BA) was condensed from CT into a stand-alone intervention. It emphasizes the relationship between activity and mood, and the importance of withdrawal and avoidance to the maintenance of depression. BA strategies include scheduling, self-monitoring, rating the degree of pleasure and achievement during daily activities, and exploring alternative behaviours with techniques such as role-playing [19]. To illustrate, consider two depressed, hospitalized cancer patients. One remains in bed, alone in the dark. The other is patting a therapy dog, borrowing a book from the volunteer or walking around the ward with an empathic relative. BA is based on the assumption that the withdrawn, isolated person will feel more depressed and the behaviourally activated patient less so.

In one randomized controlled trial, BA was as efficacious as antidepressants in severe major depression and both were superior to CT in this subgroup [20]. This suggests that BA is an alternative to medication in severely depressed patients. In a two-year follow-up, BA had similar relapse rates to CT, or continuing with an antidepressant. Both BA and CT had significantly less relapse than discontinuing an antidepressant [20]. Thus, BA may have particular applications to more severely depressed patients, with comorbid cancer, for whom cognitive reframing seems burdensome or in whom antidepressants are not well tolerated. Although specific psycho-oncology data for BA is lacking at this time, it would seem a likely area for future research.

Interpersonal Therapy

Interpersonal therapy (IPT) offers benefit to depression amelioration via its focus on interpersonal conflicts, life transitions, grief, losses and social isolation, all of which are pertinent contextual issues for the depressed cancer patient. In a meta-analysis, IPT was superior to placebo in 8/13 studies [21], but unlike CBT it had no documented additive effect when given together with an antidepressant [22]. Specific psycho-oncology data is lacking at this time, but face validity and previously cited general efficacy data suggest its utility in this setting.

Systemic Psychotherapies

Issues and Settings

The distress of cancer reverberates through couples, families and communities. Higher rates of depression have been observed in the spouses of patients with prostate cancer [23] and with non-gender based metastatic cancers [24]. This reality highlights the need for models of psychotherapy within oncology that target couples and families, especially in the setting of advanced disease. For others who may be more isolated, a group approach can be crucial as a primary means to foster social support.

Couple Therapy

The needs, goals and coping responses of patients and their close partners are highly correlated and reciprocally interdependent [25]. Relationship enhancement and protection against relational distress are the main targets of couple therapy in the oncology setting. Fostering open communication promotes mastery, while using the relationship as a key source of mutual support [26]. In the breast cancer setting, a randomized controlled trial of an active coping intervention for couples relative to usual care showed a reduction in women's depressive symptoms up to six months post treatment [27]. Couple therapy in prostate cancer is illustrated by the FOCUS intervention, which targets *F*amily involvement, *O*ptimistic attitude, *C*oping effectiveness, *U*ncertainty reduction and *S*ymptom management [28]. Spouses improved their quality of life and reduced hopelessness, likely gaining some protection against depressive outcome. Couple therapy helps achieve an adaptive adjustment when body image changes (e.g. mastectomy, colostomy, ileal conduit, limb amputation), sexuality is affected (e.g. erectile dysfunction after prostate cancer, dyspareunia after gynaecological cancers), infertility results (e.g. chemotherapy, castration surgery), issues of shame, guilt, doubt, despair or depression arise and the partner is a prime source of support.

Couple therapy in the setting of advanced cancer shifts the emphasis to anticipated loss, caregiving and existential concerns [29]. Depression was reduced through emotion-focused couple therapy that seeks to address threats to emotional engagement by recognizing distancing interactions and promoting closeness, despite the separation anxiety associated with the potential loss of a key attachment figure [30]. Effective mutual support results when couples are securely attached to each other; separation protest can take the pattern of demand-withdraw for the distressed couple, leading to disengagement and diminished safety that places some at risk. Couple therapy that identifies existential fears and supports intimacy in the face of death can do much to harness resilience and protect against demoralization and depression.

Group Therapy

Supportive-expressive group therapy (SEGT) has demonstrated efficacy in relieving distress [31, 32], and successfully aids in the treatment of depression, as well as preventing its onset in the advanced cancer setting [33]. Other models of biobehavioural group intervention have also alleviated distress [34, 35].

In cognitive-existential group therapy (CEGT) with early stage cancers, therapists aim to promote a supportive environment, facilitate grief work over the multiple losses, alter maladaptive cognitive patterns, enhance problem solving and coping skills, foster a sense of mastery and encourage review of lifestyle priorities for the future [36]. Larger groups of 10–12 patients meet weekly for 90 minutes, with careful preparation to guide expectations and more open boundaries that not only allow but encourage patient contact socially outside of the group room. Therapists strive for a clear focus on (a) the cancer journey; (b) its existential challenges; (c) coping with anti-cancer treatments; (d) supporting adherence to the medical regimen; (e) cognitive strategies to counter fear of recurrence and living with uncertainty; (f) optimizing relationships with physicians, partners, families and friends; and (g) meaning-making through recognition of what is fulfilling, creative and purposeful in life.

The goals of SEGT are to build bonds, express emotions, detoxify death, redefine life's priorities, fortify families and friends, enhance doctor-patient relationships and improve coping [37]. In placing a major emphasis on relationships, SEGT cultivates substantial meaning and purpose in living which, in turn, has a protective effect in countering depression and anxiety and ameliorating physical symptoms. The unmitigated focus on illness and potential for death transforms the group's existential ambivalence into its focus on creative living, resulting in a mature group process with prominent humour, celebration, assertiveness, altruism, community involvement, group-as-a-whole activities and eventually courageous dying. With such extraordinary influence on the cancer patient's life, it was not surprising to see SEGT actually protect cancer patients from developing new cases of clinical depression compared to those receiving usual cancer care [38].

Family Therapy

Resilience models of family-centred care that harness areas of competence, affirm skills and name capacities for growth serve to promote hope and reintegration at a time when cancer experiences can otherwise contribute to a sense of families feeling overwhelmed or hopeless [39]. Central to understanding the contribution of the family to depression in the setting of cancer is the demonstration of the high correlation between poor family functioning and relapse of depression [40] or the development of complicated grief [41], resulting eventually in a morbid bereavement outcome [42].

In a randomized controlled trial targeting 'at risk' families, family therapy that aimed to optimize family functioning through promotion of effective communication, enhanced cohesion and adaptive resolution of conflict was shown to reduce depression and support mourning arising from family loss due to cancer [43]. The more pronounced the relational dysfunction, the greater the number of family sessions that are needed across the bereavement phase. In general, mild family dysfunction can be aided by four to six sessions, whereas 10–12 sessions may be needed for those with pronounced dysfunction. Openness to discussion of death and dying and early containment of conflict prove beneficial until improved communication and closeness help family members to tolerate any differences of opinion [44]. Therapists make use of circular questions to reveal family dynamics and offer regular summaries as a means to help families integrate understanding of their patterns of relating and coping with loss and change [45]. Commencing therapy when the cancer patient is still alive and present to voice his or her opinions establishes a model of family care that is preventive, cost-effective and enables continuity of support to be carried into bereavement.

Systemic therapies, delivered in the setting of a cancer patient or family member suffering from depression, nurture a supportive environment, attend to relevant perpetuating influences and ensure that the couple, family and community are harnessed as therapeutic agents to assist in the active treatment of the depression. Couple and group models are important in early stage and survivorship settings, while family therapy comes to the fore with advanced cancers.

PSYCHOTHERAPIES IN ADVANCED CANCER AND PALLIATIVE CARE

Psychological well-being is inevitably challenged in individuals with advanced disease, because of the profound and diverse stresses and burdens associated with it. These invariably include physical suffering and disability, the threat of impending mortality, dramatic alterations in support needs and personal relationships, the challenge of navigat-

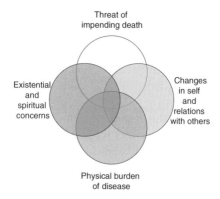

Figure 8.1 The inter-related challenges of terminal disease.

ing a complex healthcare system and making treatment decisions that have life and death implications (see Figure 8.1). Depressive symptoms in individuals with advanced disease may best be understood as a final common pathway of distress in response to these multiple individual, social and disease-related risk factors [46].

Early interventions to address the challenges of advanced disease and to treat depressive symptoms may help to protect or improve emotional well-being and quality of life. Unfortunately, however, the majority of patients at this stage of disease who suffer from clinically significant depression are not referred for psychosocial or psychiatric care and most of those referred do not receive specific or adequate treatment for depression [47]. Although routine distress screening is now regarded as a standard in cancer care at all stages of the disease [48–50], its benefit has been limited by the relative failure of cancer treatment centres to provide effective interventions that follow from such screening [51].

The alleviation and treatment of depression in individuals with advanced cancer requires an integrated approach, which includes attention to symptom control, the social environment and the psychological disturbance itself. Psychological treatments for depression are preferred by patients with advanced cancer compared to pharmacological ones [52]; and the format of individual or couple psychotherapy often becomes most appropriate as the disease progresses. Individual sessions not only permit the content of therapy to be flexibly tailored to address specific individual needs, but the timing of the sessions can also be more easily adjusted to take into account other clinic appointments, investigations and treatments, and the frequent fluctuations in health status at this stage of disease [53–55]. Psycho-therapeutic treatment of this kind is best initiated before debilitating physical symptoms or cognitive impairment limit the capacity for engagement and self-reflection. Further, the potential for unpredict-able clinical deterioration requires that the goals of treatment be accomplished in a relatively brief period of time.

Many individual psychotherapeutic modalities used to treat depres-sion in early stage cancer have utility for patients with advanced disease, with greater emphasis on existential and loss-related themes. Models of therapy include logotherapy, existential psychotherapy, grief therapy, life review, life narrative and interpersonal therapy [56]. The research that has been conducted thus far to investigate the effectiveness of individual psychotherapies for the treatment of depression in patients with advanced disease has been limited by methodological problems, such as the absence of appropriate inclusion criteria for the severity of depression and inadequate description of the methods of randomization [52, 57]. Also, several individual psychotherapy inter-ventions are currently being investigated to determine their effective-ness in the treatment of depression in patients with advanced disease. These treatments can be broadly categorized into those that promote active coping strategies and those that emphasize the communication and understanding of emotional experience and the joint creation of meaning, usually described as supportive-expressive therapies.

Interventions to Promote Active Coping Strategies

These interventions include behaviourally-focused therapies, such as relaxation therapy [58], biofeedback, guided imagery and hypno-sis [59, 60], as well as CBT directed toward ameliorating dysfunc-tional cognitions [61, 62] and problem-solving therapy [63–66].

Savard *et al.* [61] reported a randomized trial of CBT with a wait list control in 45 women with metastatic cancer and depression based on Hospital Anxiety and Depression Scale - Depression (HADS-D) scores of 7 or Beck Depression Inventory (BDI) scores of 15 or more;

they found significant reductions in depression scores. More recently, Moorey *et al.* [66] reported findings from a cluster randomized controlled trial of CBT for depression delivered by specially trained nurses in which 80 patients with advanced cancer and HADS scores of 8 or more on either the anxiety or depression subscale entered the trial. They found a significant treatment effect for anxiety, but not for depression. Further research with larger sample sizes is needed to determine more conclusively the benefit of CBT for the treatment of depression in this population.

Problem-solving therapy may be particularly relevant in the treatment of patients with advanced cancer with regard to the problems associated with progressive disability, dependency, end of life planning, and the anticipated burden on loved ones [67–69], and it has been found to be highly acceptable to patients [65]. Two large, recently conducted randomized controlled trials have found this therapy to be effective in reducing depressive symptoms in patients with cancer [63, 64], although the intervention was not specifically designed for advanced cancer patients. In the trial reported by Strong *et al.* [64], 16% of the 101 initial intervention participants had metastatic disease and in the Ell *et al.* trial [63], 28% of the 242 initial intervention participants had Stage III, IV or recurrent disease. However, a noteworthy strength of these interventions, and to some extent of the CBT interventions, is that they occurred within a collaborative care context, making coordinated and optimal use of existing institutional infrastructure and health professionals [70].

Collaborative care has been recommended to address the inadequacy of depression care in patients with cancer and other chronic medical conditions [71], due to the failure to detect depression, to provide an evidence-based treatment, and to actively monitor and modify patient responses to treatment [72]. Elements of collaborative care incorporated into problem-solving therapy include the use of clinic distress screening to identify depressed patients [64], communication with primary care doctors and oncologists about the patients' depressive symptoms [64], use of trained health professionals from social work, nursing and psychiatry in the delivery of manualized psychosocial and pharmacological treatment [63, 64], patient monitoring after treatment ends [63, 64], and assistance with navigating and accessing community services [63]. The use of social workers and nurses in the delivery of problem-solving therapy also increases the feasibility of the interventions in institutions with limited resources and staffing for psychosocial care.

Supportive-Expressive, Narrative and Existential Therapies

These are therapies focused on emotional modulation, self-under-standing, the facilitation of reflective functioning and promotion of psychological growth [73]. Such interventions allow individuals to process intensely painful affect states that have been evoked by the trauma of diagnosis, recurrence and progression of disease and by the multiple losses that have occurred and are anticipated. The increased awareness of mortality and the dramatic alterations in the assumptive world of those with advanced disease paradoxically create a 'now moment' in which the capacity for authentic and deep engagement in the treatment process is often heightened. The empathic engagement of the supportive-expressive therapist and the creation of a reflective space within the treatment may provide a profound experience of support and allow the joint creation of narrative meaning about the patient's life trajectory and illness experience. Such treatments also facilitate the renegotiation of attachment relationships and the reso-lution of grief and mourning which may be associated with persistent depressive symptoms.

Dignity therapy and CALM (Managing Cancer And Living Mean-ingfully) therapy are two examples of supportive-expressive therapies designed specifically for patients with advanced disease to target depressive symptoms and other manifestations of suffering and distress. Both are semi-structured interventions which target the underlying problems and challenges associated with advanced and terminal disease.

Dignity Therapy

Dignity therapy is a brief individual therapy designed to address psychosocial and existential distress in patients near the end of life [74]. It was developed from the perspective that dignity, or the sense that one's life has been and continues to be worthwhile, is fundamentally challenged in palliative populations, and that the protection of dignity is central to psychological well-being.

Dignity is considered to include such themes as generativity and continuity of self, maintenance of pride and hope, role preservation, alleviation of concerns about the burden to others and the aftermath, and about the tenor or quality of care that is received [56]. The dignity model was empirically-derived from evidence of a strong association between the experience of undermined dignity and symptoms of depression, anxiety, the desire for death, demoralization, the sense of burden to others, and poorer quality of life [75].

The dignity therapy interview framework includes questions related to the above content themes. The initial interviewer prompt is: 'Tell me a little about your life history, particularly the parts that you either remember most or think were most important'. Therapists are then encouraged to follow patient cues and shape the interview based on patient interest and response. The goal is to have patients describe the aspects of their lives of which they are proudest, what is most meaningful to them, what they want to be remembered for, and/or what they want to share with loved ones. The therapeutic stance is inquisitive, helping patients to structure and organize their thoughts, as well as empathic and nonjudgmental. Designed to be brief and potentially provided at the bedside, there are usually only one to three sessions of 30 to 60 minutes length required. These are audio-taped, transcribed and edited. A resulting 'generativity document' is returned to patients to leave to a family member or friend.

A pre-post design study found that dignity therapy improved depressive symptoms in patients with a life expectancy of less than six months, the majority of whom had cancer [74], and lessened the suffering and distress in their terminally ill relatives [76]. An international, multicentre randomized trial is currently underway to further test this intervention in palliative care settings [77].

CALM Therapy

CALM is a brief, individual psychotherapy model, currently undergoing testing, that is designed to address the specific problems and risk factors that contribute to depressive symptoms [46] in patients with advanced disease, but with a life expectancy of more than six months. CALM is rooted in several broad theoretical traditions, including relational theory, attachment theory, and existential psychotherapy. It shares many features in common with manualized supportive-expressive [32, 78–84], cognitive-existential [85, 86], and meaning-centred [87] group psychotherapies developed for patients with advanced and terminal disease. It provides support for symptom management and navigation of the health care system, and a reflective space which allows for the processing of thoughts and emotions, and the consideration of practical and existential questions. CALM was designed not only to relieve depression and other forms of distress, but also to promote psychological growth, which has been suggested may be possible at this stage of disease [88]. To enhance its effectiveness, CALM is embedded within a collaborative care context, modelled on interventions which have been shown to be effective in reducing depressive symptoms in mixed cancer [63, 64] and other medical populations [89, 90].

CALM therapy consists of three to six individual sessions delivered over three months, with two booster sessions offered in the subsequent three months. It comprises four empirically derived modules or domains of concern [46], which serve as a framework to address the common and inter-related stressors which face patients with advanced cancer (see Figure 8.1). The time devoted to each module or domain varies, based on the needs and concerns of the individual patient, as determined in the first session, which consists of a psychosocial assessment and an introduction and discussion of the modules with the patient. Sessions proceed by addressing individual issues in order from most to least important. The modules are laid out in Table 8.2, covering their key themes, goals for each module, relevant therapist activities and the main outcomes worked towards within each module.

Research has consistently highlighted that symptom management and effective relationships with healthcare providers, including clear communication, contribution to decision-making and individualized care, are major concerns for patients facing advanced disease and the end of life [91–93]. Key attention to optimal symptom management is therefore imperative for other aspects of psychotherapeutic work to proceed [94].

Table 8.2 Modules for Managing Cancer And Living Meaningfully (CALM) therapy

Module	Goal	Therapist activity	Outcomes
Symptom management and communication with health care providers	To explore the experience of symptoms and to support active engagement in treatment and disease management, together with collaborative relationships with health care providers	Therapists work to maintain a balanced patient perspective, and to act as an advocate between the patient and other caregivers	Improved adherence to symptom management regimens; improved teamwork; better coordination of care; clearer agreement about the goals of care
Changes in self and relations with close others	To address any damage to the sense of self and alterations in social and intimate relationships that are imposed by advanced disease	Provide couple or family sessions to explore relational dynamics, to assist with disruptions in the relational equilibrium and to prepare for the challenges and tasks that lie ahead	Better understanding and consensus about the goals of care; improved relational communication, cohesion and mutual support

Spirituality or sense of meaning and purpose	To explore the patient's spiritual beliefs and/or sense of meaning and purpose in life in the face of suffering and advanced disease	Therapists can facilitate and support meaning-making as an adaptive strategy to manage a situation which is often otherwise experienced as beyond one's personal control	Validation and/or reevaluation of priorities and goals; facilitation of an active approach to the end of life experience
Thinking of the future, hope and mortality	To explore anticipatory fears and anxieties and provide forum for discussion of life closure and death preparation activities	Normalize anxieties regarding dying and death; support open communication about the future and planning	Acceptance of agreed goals of care; a balance between tasks of living and dying

Increased dependency, and role and identity changes are common experiences of the advanced cancer patient. An individual's expectations of social support and his capacity to make use of this support, reflected in his attachment style [95, 96], have been shown to modulate the emergence or expression of distress [97]. Practical issues such as the household division of labour, financial responsibilities and parenting roles intersect with a variety of relational themes connected to attachment security, intimacy and emotional communication. As one CALM patient expressed, 'sometimes friends change and disappear, even best friends when one is ill, because they don't understand what you are feeling or what to do'. The timing and nature of disclosure to children and other family members about the prognosis and how to support them through the illness process are also commonly addressed.

Existential issues (i.e. spirituality, meaning and purpose) are often of increased importance near the end of life [98]. In the medically ill, meaning, purpose in life and faith have been found to be inversely correlated with depression [99]. For some, the crisis of illness and dying may strengthen long held religious or philosophical views. For others, unanswerable questions such as 'why me?', 'what comes next?', or 'why must my family suffer?' trigger distress and challenge existing beliefs. Consistent with Yalom [100], the working through of these issues leads to reevaluation of priorities and life goals and/or the methods for their achievement. The treatment allows patients in this circumstance to focus not only on the end, which is approaching, but on the life which can be lived [101].

Research has shown that patients and families consistently identify advance care planning, life closure and death preparation activities as important components of a positive dying experience [92, 93]. Further, evidence confirms that patients and families facing advanced and terminal disease welcome the frank, but empathic, discussion of such issues and that hope is more likely to be sustained when it is not based on false expectations [94]. Indeed, the opportunity to speak openly of dying and death, and the normalization or 'detoxification' of anxieties associated with these outcomes can be profoundly validating and paradoxically calming [78, 79]. One CALM patient compared his experience of advancing disease to that of being in an old Western movie, specifically of being caught in the 'enclosing circle' of a wagon train, in which he was 'running out of ammunition' with 'more people coming to attack'. He said that he knew that 'there is not going to be a happy ending' but that the therapy was helping him to 'take advantage of the time available'.

Suicidality and the Desire to Hasten Death

Depression towards the end of life has been strongly associated with development of a desire to hasten death, which can present as a request for suicide [102–104]. Indeed, rates of suicide increase at this phase of life in the context of poorly controlled pain and depression, unrecognized demoralization and poor family support. Suicidal thinking typically fluctuates with poor symptom control, including poor control of depressive symptoms.

The resultant psychotherapeutic approach is coordinated alongside excellent symptom management, antidepressant medication, a narrative approach to understanding who this person is and what sources of meaning and fulfilment have been present in his/her life, a family-centred approach to rallying support and care for the patient, and continuity of care that focuses on reconnecting with sources of continued meaning, affirmation of the person and nurturance of hope for the life that remains.

CONCLUSIONS

Challenges exist with patients struggling with chronic, relapsing or unremitting depressive and dysthymic states. Careful attention to integrated care provision, coordination of pharmacological and psychotherapeutic therapies, and consideration of unrecognized perpetuating factors (be they poorly controlled physical symptoms with disease progression, unaddressed systemic issues, confounding spiritual or social issues, drug interactions, or direct tumour effects via cytokines or paraneoplastic processes) are vital as the treatment team journeys with its patients and their illnesses.

Depression increases suffering in the oncology setting. A broad range of therapies now exist to ameliorate this distress. The art of such therapy is the strategic and, indeed, eclectic selection of components from several models to best respond to the needs of the individual patient and his/her family in the specific circumstances, whether clinical, psychological, spiritual or social. Although we have pragmatically placed more emphasis on CBT in early cancer and supportive-expressive therapies in advanced cancer, clearly the wise therapist selects whatever model offers most to the needs of the patient at that time. Existential, spiritual and meaning-based themes are commonly met and dealt with in the early stage patient with cancer. Also, many of these therapies are appropriately combined with psychotropic medication.

Several meta-analyses have been conducted that confirm the effectiveness of psychotherapy in assuaging depression in patients with cancer [9, 12, 15, 16]. Relief of demoralization and despair is a crucial feature of whole-person and family-centred care, delivered in pursuit of enriching quality of life and helping sustain worthwhile living right through to the final moment when death intervenes.

REFERENCES

1. Jacobsen, P.B. and Jim, H.S. (2008) Psychosocial interventions for anxiety and depression in adult cancer patients: achievements and challenges. *CA Cancer J. Clin.*, **58**, 214–230.

2. American Psychiatric Association (2000) *Diagnostic and Statistical Manual of Mental Disorders*, 4th edn, text revision, American Psychiatric Association, Washington.

3. Clay, S., Allen, J. and Parran, T. (2008) A review of addiction. *Postgrad. Med.*, **120**, E01–E07.

4. Beck, A.T. (1964) Thinking and depression II: theory and therapy. *Arch. Gen. Psychiatry*, **10**, 561–571.

5. Beck, J. (1995) *Cognitive Therapy: Basics and Beyond*, Guilford, New York.

6. Beck, A.T., Rush, A.J., Shaw, B.F. and Emery, G. (1979) *Cognitive Therapy of Depression*, Guilford, New York.

7. Spitzer, R., Kroenke, K. and Williams, J. (1999) Validation and utility of a self-report version of PRIME-MD: the PHQ primary care study. Primary Care Evaluation of Mental Disorders. Patient Health Questionnaire. *JAMA*, **282**, 1737–1744.

8. White, C.A. (2001) *Cognitive Behaviour Therapy for Chronic Medical Problems. A Guide to Assessment and Treatment in Practice*, Wiley, Chichester.

9. Osborn, R., Demoncada, A. and Feuerstein, M. (2006) Psychosocial interventions for depression, anxiety, and quality of life in cancer survivors: meta-analyses. *Int. J. Psychiatry Med.*, **36**, 13–34.

10. Sheard, T. and Maguire, P. (1999) The effect of psychological interventions on anxiety and depression in cancer patients: results of two meta-analyses. *Br. J. Cancer*, **80**, 1770–1780.

11. Pitceathly, C., Maguire, P., Fletcher, I. *et al.* (2009) Can a brief psychological intervention prevent anxiety or depressive disorders in cancer patients? A randomized controlled trial. *Ann. Oncol.*, **20**, 928–934.

12. Nezu, A.M., Maguth Nezu, C., Friedman, S.H. *et al.* (1998) *Helping Cancer Patients Cope. A Problem Solving Approach*, American Psychological Association, Washington.

13. Nezu, A., Nezu, C.M., Felgoise, S. *et al.* (2003) Project Genesis: assessing the efficacy of problem-solving therapy for distressed adult cancer patients. *J. Consult. Clin. Psychol.*, **71**, 1036–1048.

14. Devine, E.C. and Westlake, S.K. (2003) Meta-analysis of the effect of psychoeducational interventions on pain in adults with cancer. *Oncol. Nurs. Forum*, **30**, 75–89.

15. Barsevick, A., Sweeney, C., Haney, E. and Chung, E. (2002) A systematic qualitative analysis of psychoeducational interventions for depression in patients with cancer. *Oncol. Nurs. Forum*, **29**, 73–84.

16. Wells, K.J., Battaglia, T.A., Dudley, D.J. *et al.* (2008) Patient navigation: state of the art or is it science? *Cancer*, **113**, 1999–2010.

17. Luebbert, K., Dahme, B. and Hasenbring, M. (2001) The effectiveness of relaxation training in reducing treatment-related symptoms and improving emotional adjustment in acute non-surgical cancer treatment: a meta-analytical review. *Psychooncology*, **10**, 490–502.

18. Jacobsen, P.B., Meade, C.D., Stein, K.D. *et al.* (2002) Efficacy and costs of two forms of stress management training for cancer patients undergoing chemotherapy. *J. Clin. Oncol.*, **20**, 2851–2862.

19. Dimidjian, S., Hollon, S.D., Dobson, K.S. *et al.* (2006) Randomized trial of behavioral activation, cognitive therapy, and antidepressant

medication in the acute treatment of adults with major depression. *J. Consult. Clin. Psychol.*, **74**, 658–670.

20. Dobson, K.S., Hollon, S.D., Dimidjian, S. *et al.* (2008) Randomized trial of behavioral activation, cognitive therapy, and antidepressant medication in the prevention of relapse and recurrence in major depression. *J. Consult. Clin. Psychol.*, **76**, 468–477.

21. de Mello, M., de Jesus Mari, J., Bacaltchuk, J. *et al.* (2005) A systematic review of research findings on the efficacy of interpersonal therapy for depressive disorders. *Eur. Arch. Psychiatry Clin. Neurosci.*, **255**, 75–82.

22. Lesperance, F., Frasure-Smith, N., Koszycki, D. *et al.* (2007) Effects of citalopram and interpersonal psychotherapy on depression in patients with coronary artery disease: the Canadian Cardiac Randomized Evaluation of Antidepressant and Psychotherapy Efficacy (CREATE) trial. *JAMA*, **297**, 367–379.

23. Couper, J.W., Bloch, S., Love, A. *et al.* (2006) The psychosocial impact of prostate cancer on patients and their partners. *Med. J. Australia*, **185**, 428–432.

24. Braun, M., Mikulincer, M., Rydall, A. *et al.* (2007) Hidden morbidity in cancer: spouse caregivers. *J. Clin. Oncol.*, **25**, 4829–4834.

25. Hagedoorn, M., Sanderman, R., Bolks, H.N. *et al.* (2008) Distress in couples coping with cancer: a meta-analysis and critical review of role and gender effects. *Psychol. Bull.*, **134**, 1–30.

26. Lepore, S.J., Ragan, J.D. and Jones, S. (2000) Talking facilitates cognitive-emotional processes of adaptation to an acute stressor. *J. Pers. Soc. Psychol.*, **78**, 499–508.

27. Manne, S.L., Ostroff, J.S., Winkel, G. *et al.* (2005) Couple-focused group intervention for women with early stage breast cancer. *J. Consult. Clin. Psychol.*, **73**, 634–646.

28. Northouse, L.L., Mood, D.W., Schafenacker, A. *et al.* (2007) Randomized clinical trial of a family intervention for prostate cancer patients and their spouses. *Cancer*, **110**, 2809–2818.

29. McLean, L.M. and Jones, J.M. (2007) A review of distress and its management in couples facing end-of-life cancer. *Psychooncology*, **16**, 603–616.

30. McLean, L.M. and Nissim, R. (2007) Marital therapy for couples facing advanced cancer: case review. *Palliat. Support. Care*, **5**, 303–313.

31. Classen, C., Butler, L.D., Koopman, C. *et al.* (2001) Supportive-expressive group therapy and distress in patients with metastatic breast

cancer: a randomized clinical intervention trial. *Arch. Gen. Psychiatry*, **58**, 494–501.

32. Goodwin, P.J., Leszcz, M., Ennis, M. *et al.* (2001) The effect of group psychosocial support on survival in metastatic breast cancer. *N. Engl. J. Med.*, **345**, 1719–1726.

33. Kissane, D.W., Grabsch, B., Clarke, D.M. *et al.* (2007) Supportive-expressive group therapy for women with metastatic breast cancer: survival and psychosocial outcome from a randomized controlled trial. *Psychooncology*, **16**, 227–286.

34. Andersen, B.L., Farrar, W.B., Golden-Kreutz, D. *et al.* (2007) Distress reduction from a psychological intervention contributes to improved health for cancer patients. *Brain Behav. Immunol.*, 21, 953–961.

35. Edelman, S., Bell, D.R. and Kidman, A.D. (1999) A group cognitive behaviour therapy programme with metastatic breast cancer patients. *Psychooncology*, **8**, 306–314.

36. Kissane, D.W., Bloch, S., Miach, P. *et al.* (1997) Cognitive-existential group therapy for patients with primary breast cancer – techniques and themes. *Psychooncology*, **6**, 25–33.

37. Spiegel, D. and Classen, C. (2000) *Group Therapy for Cancer Patients. A Research-Based Handbook of Psychological Care*, Basic Books, New York.

38. Kissane, D.W., Grabsch, B., Clarke, D.M. *et al.* (2004) Supportive-expressive group therapy: the transformation of existential ambivalence into creative living while enhancing adherence to anti-cancer therapies. *Psychooncology*, **13**, 755–768.

39. Zaider, T. and Kissane, D.W. (2007) Resilient families, in *Resilience in Palliative Care* (eds B. Monroe and D. Oliviere), Oxford University Press, Oxford, pp. 67–81.

40. Keitner, G.I. and Miller, I.W. (1990) Family functioning and major depression: an overview. *Am. J. Psychiatry*, **147**, 1128–1137.

41. Kissane, D.W., Bloch, S., Burns, W.I. *et al.* (1994) Perceptions of family functioning and cancer. *Psychooncology*, **3**, 259–269.

42. Kissane, D.W., Bloch, S., Dowe, D.L. *et al.* (1996) The Melbourne family grief study, I: perceptions of family functioning in bereavement. *Am. J. Psychiatry*, **153**, 650–658.

43. Kissane, D.W., McKenzie, M., Bloch, S. *et al.* (2006) Family focused grief therapy: a randomized, controlled trial in palliative care and bereavement. *Am. J. Psychiatry*, **163**, 1208–1218.

44. Kissane, D.W. and Bloch, S. (2002) *Family Focused Grief Therapy: A Model of Family-Centered Care During Palliative Care and Bereavement*, Open University Press, Buckingham.

45. Dumont, I. and Kissane, D.W. (2009) Techniques for framing questions in conducting family meetings in palliative care. *Palliat. Support. Care*, **7**, 163–170.

46. Rodin, G., Lo, C., Mikulincer, M. *et al.* (2009) Pathways to distress: the multiple determinants of depression, hopelessness and the desire for hastened death in metastatic cancer patients. *Soc. Sci. Med.*, **68**, 562–569.

47. Ellis, J., Lin, J., Walsh, A. *et al.* (2009) Predictors of referral for specialized psychosocial oncology care in patients with metastatic cancer: the contributions of age, distress, and marital status. *J. Clin. Oncol.*, **27**, 699–705.

48. NCCN (2009) *Clinical Practice Guidelines in Oncology: Distress Management, Version 1. 2010*, National Comprehensive Cancer Network, Washington.

49. NICE (2004) *NICE Guidance on Cancer Services. Improving Supportive and Palliative Care for Adults with Cancer: The Manual*, National Institute for Clinical Excellence, London.

50. Turner, J., Zapart, S., Pedersen, K. *et al.* (2005) Clinical practice guidelines for the psychosocial care of adults with cancer. *Psychooncology*, **14**, 159–173.

51. Jacobsen, P.B. (2009) Promoting evidence-based psychosocial care for cancer patients. *Psychooncology*, **18**, 6–13.

52. Akechi, T., Okuyama, T., Onishi, J. *et al.* (2008) Psychotherapy for depression among incurable cancer patients. *Cochrane Database Syst. Rev.*, **2**, CD005537.

53. Edelman, S., Bell, D.R. and Kidman, A.D. (1999) A group cognitive behavior therapy programme with metastatic breast cancer patients. *Psychooncology*, **8**, 295–305.

54. Clark, M.M., Bostwick, J.M. and Rummans, T.A. (2003) Group and individual treatment strategies for distress in cancer patients. *Mayo Clin. Proc.*, **78**, 1538–1543.

55. Sherman, A.C., Pennington, J., Latif, U. *et al.* (2007) Patient preferences regarding cancer group psychotherapy interventions: a view from the inside. *Psychosomatics*, **48**, 426–432.

56. Chochinov, H.M., Hack, T., Hassard, T. *et al.* (2004) Dignity and psychotherapeutic considerations in end-of-life care. *J. Palliat. Care*, **20**, 134–142.

57. Rodin, G., Lloyd, N., Katz, M. *et al.* (2007) The treatment of depression in cancer patients: a systematic review. *Support. Care Cancer*, **15**, 123–136.

58. Sloman, R. (2002) Relaxation and imagery for anxiety and depression control in community patients with advanced cancer. *Cancer Nurs.*, **25**, 432–435.

59. Laidlaw, T., Bennett, B.M., Dwivedi, P. *et al.* (2005) Quality of life and mood changes in metastatic breast cancer after training in self-hypnosis or Johrei: a short report. *Contemp. Hypnosis*, **22**, 84–93.

60. Liossi, C. (2006) Hypnosis in cancer care. *Contemp. Hypnosis*, **23**, 47–57.

61. Savard, J., Simard, S., Giguere, I. *et al.* (2006) Randomized clinical trial of cognitive therapy for depression in women with metastatic breast cancer: psychological and immunological effects. *Palliat. Support. Care*, **4**, 219–237.

62. Levesque, M., Savard, J., Simard, S. *et al.* (2004) Efficacy of cognitive therapy for depression among women with metastatic cancer: a single-case experimental study. *J. Behav. Ther. Exp. Psychiatry*, **35**, 287–305.

63. Ell, K., Xie, B., Quon, B. *et al.* (2008) Randomized controlled trial of collaborative care management of depression among low-income patients with cancer. *J. Clin. Oncol.*, **26**, 4488–4496.

64. Strong, V., Waters, R., Hibberd, C. *et al.* (2008) Management of depression for people with cancer (SMaRT oncology 1): a randomized trial. *Lancet*, **372**, 40–48.

65. Wood, B.C. and Mynors-Wallis, L.M. (1997) Problem-solving therapy in palliative care. *Palliative Med.*, **11**, 49–54.

66. Moorey, S., Cort, E., Kapari, M. *et al.* (2009) A cluster randomized controlled trial of cognitive behaviour therapy for common mental disorders in patients with advanced cancer. *Psychol. Med.*, **39**, 713–723.

67. Chochinov, H.M., Tartaryn, D.J., Wilson, K.G. *et al.* (2000) Prognostic awareness and the terminally ill. *Psychosomatics*, **41**, 500–504.

68. Tan, A., Zimmermann, C. and Rodin, G. (2005) Interpersonal processes in palliative care: an attachment perspective on the patient-clinician relationship. *Palliative Med.*, **39**, 143–150.

69. McPherson, C.J., Wilson, K.G. and Murray, M.A. (2007) Feeling like a burden to others: a systematic review focusing on the end of life. *Palliative Med.*, **21**, 115–128.

70. Walker, J. and Sharpe, M. (2009) Depression care for people with cancer: a collaborative care intervention. *Gen. Hosp. Psychiatry*, **31**, 436–441.

71. Sharpe, M., Strong, V., Allen, K. *et al.* (2004) Major depression in outpatients attending a regional cancer centre: screening and unmet treatment needs. *Br. J. Cancer*, **90**, 314–320.

72. Greenberg, D.B. (2004) Barriers to the treatment of depression in cancer patients. *J. Natl. Cancer Inst. Monogr.*, **32**, 127–135.

73. Rodin, G. (2009) Individual psychotherapy for the patient with advanced disease, in *Handbook of Psychiatry in Palliative Medicine* (eds H. Chochinov and W. Breitbart), Oxford University Press, London, pp. 443–453.

74. Chochinov, H.M., Hack, T., Hassard, T. *et al.* (2005) Dignity therapy: a novel psychotherapeutic intervention for patients near the end of life. *J. Clin. Oncol.*, **23**, 5520–5525.

75. Chochinov, H.M., Hack, T., Hassard, T. *et al.* (2002) Dignity in the terminally ill: a cross-sectional, cohort study. *Lancet*, **360**, 2026–2030.

76. McClement, S., Chochinov, H., Hack, T. *et al.* (2007) Dignity therapy: family member perspectives. *J. Palliat. Med.*, **10**, 1076–1082.

77. Hall, S., Edmonds, P., Harding, R. *et al.* (2009) Assessing the feasibility, acceptability, and potential effectiveness of Dignity Therapy for people with advanced cancer referred to a hospital-based palliative care team: study protocol. *BMC Palliat. Care*, **8**, 5.

78. Spiegel, D., Bloom, J.R. and Yalom, I. (1981) Group support for patients with metastatic cancer: a randomized outcome study. *Arch. Gen. Psychiatry*, **38**, 527–533.

79. Spiegel, D., Morrow, G.R., Classen, C. *et al.* (1999) Group psychotherapy for recently diagnosed breast cancer patients: a multicenter feasibility study. *Psychooncology*, **8**, 482–493.

80. Classen, C., Butler, L.D., Koopman, C. *et al.* (2001) Supportive-expressive group therapy and distress in patients with metastatic breast cancer: a randomized clinical intervention trial. *Arch. Gen. Psychiatry*, **58**, 494–501.

81. Giese-Davis, J., Koopman, C., Butler, L.D. *et al.* (2002) Change in emotion-regulation strategy for women with metastatic breast cancer following supportive-expressive group therapy. *J. Consult. Clin. Psychol.*, **70**, 916–925.

82. Breitbart, W. (2001) Spirituality and meaning in supportive care: spirituality- and meaning-centered group psychotherapy interventions in advanced cancer. *Supp. Care Cancer*, **10**, 272–280.

83. Bordeleau, L., Szalai, J.P., Ennis, M. *et al.* (2003) Quality of life in a randomized trial of group psychosocial support in metastatic breast cancer: overall effects of the intervention and an exploration of missing data. *J. Clin. Oncol.*, **21**, 1944–1951.

84. Weiss, J.J., Mulder, C.L., Antoni, M.H. *et al.* (2003) Effects of a supportive-expressive group intervention on long-term psychosocial

adjustment in HIV-infected gay men. *Psychother. Psychosom.*, **72**, 132–140.

85. Kissane, D.W., Bloch, S., Smith, G.C. *et al.* (2003) Cognitive-existential group psychotherapy for women with primary breast cancer: a randomized controlled trial. *Psychooncology*, **12**, 532–546.

86. Kissane, D.W., Love, A., Hatton, A. *et al.* (2004) Effect of cognitive-existential group therapy on survival in early-stage breast cancer. *J. Clin. Oncol.*, **22**, 4255–4260.

87. Breitbart, W., Rosenfeld, B., Gibson, C. *et al.* (2010) Meaning-centred group psychotherapy for patients with advanced cancer: a pilot randomized controlled trial. *Psychooncology.* **19**, 21–28.

88. Block, S.D. (2001) Psychological considerations, growth, and transcendence at the end of life: the art of the possible. *JAMA*, **285**, 2898–2905.

89. Gilbody, S., Bower, P., Fletcher, J. *et al.* (2006) Collaborative care for depression: a cumulative meta-analysis and review of longer-term outcomes. *Arch. Intern. Med.*, **166**, 2314–2321.

90. Katon, W.J., Russo, J.E., Von Korff, M. *et al.* (2008) Long-term effects on medical costs of improving depression outcomes in patients with depression and diabetes. *Diabetes Care*, **31**, 1155–1159.

91. Coll, P.P., Duffy, J.D., Micholovich, E. and Cohen, S. (2002) Best practices in hospital end-of-life care. *Conn. Med.*, **66**, 671–675.

92. Howell, D. and Brazil, K. (2005) Reaching common ground: a patient-family-based conceptual framework of quality EOL care. *J. Palliat. Care*, **21**, 19–26.

93. Hales, S., Zimmermann, C. and Rodin, G. (2008) The quality of dying and death. *Arch. Intern. Med.*, **168**, 912–918.

94. Rodin, G., Mackay, J.A., Zimmermann, C. *et al.* (2009) Clinician-patient communication: a systematic review. *Support. Care Cancer*, **17**, 627–644.

95. Lo, C., Walsh, A., Mikulincer, M. *et al.* (2009) Measuring attachment security in patients with advanced cancer: psychometric properties of a modified and brief Experiences in Close Relationships scale. *Psychooncology*, **18**, 490–499.

96. Lo, C., Li, M. and Rodin, G. (2008) The assessment and treatment of distress in cancer patients: overview and future directions. *Minerva Psichiatrica*, **49**, 129–143.

97. Rodin, G., Walsh, A., Zimmermann, C. *et al.* (2007) The contribution of attachment security and social support to depressive symptoms in patients with metastatic cancer. *Psychooncology*, **16**, 1080–1091.

98. LeMay, K. and Wilson, K.G. (2008) Treatment of existential distress in life threatening illness: a review of manualized interventions. *Clin. Psychol. Rev.*, **28**, 472–493.

99. McClain, C.S., Rosenfeld, B. and Breitbart, W. (2003) Effect of spiritual well-being on end-of-life despair in terminally-ill cancer patients. *Lancet*, **362**, 1603–1607.

100. Yalom, I.D. (1980) *Existential Psychotherapy*, Basic Books, New York.

101. Rodin, G. and Zimmermann, C. (2008) Psychoanalytic reflections on mortality: a reconsideration. *J. Am. Acad. Psychoanal. Dyn. Psychiatry*, **36**, 181–196.

102. Morita, T., Kawa, M., Honke, Y. *et al.* (2004) Existential concerns of terminally ill cancer patients receiving specialized palliative care in Japan. *Support. Care Cancer*, **12** (2), 137–140.

103. Kissane, D. (2004) The contribution of demoralization to end of life decision-making. *Hastings Cent. Rep.*, **34**, 21–31.

104. Chochinov, H.M., Hack, T., Hassard, T. *et al.* (2005) Understanding the will to live in patients nearing death. *Psychosomatics*, **46**, 7–10.

CHAPTER 9

Depression and Cancer: the Role of Culture and Social Disparities

Christoffer Johansen, Susanne Oksbjerg Dalton and Pernille Envold Bidstrup

Department of Psychosocial Cancer Research, Danish Institute of Cancer Epidemiology, Danish Cancer Society, Copenhagen, Denmark

Depression is a multifactorial disorder, which is affected by gender, genetics, family environment, childhood sexual abuse, bereavement, personality, previous psychological disorders, stressful life events, low social support, substance misuse, and marital difficulties [1, 2]. The social context may also play a role in both the risk for and recognition of depression. Today, most clinicians and researchers in the field agree that social, economic and cultural factors moderate the movement from normalcy to any form of depression. Understanding the role of cultural, social and economic factors in depression is essential for prevention, as these factors are potentially modifiable.

In this chapter, we discuss the role of culture and socioeconomic status in depression and cancer. We describe the constructs of culture, ethnicity and socioeconomic position and how they are defined and measured in epidemiological health research. In several large, popu-

Depression and Cancer   Edited by David W. Kissane, Mario Maj and Norman Sartorius
© 2011 John Wiley & Sons, Ltd

lation-based, nationwide studies in Denmark, we have considered the effects of social disparity on depression and cancer in a society with equal access to healthcare. Use of these data is discussed thoroughly, and we aim to show how they can overcome some of the methodological limitations that characterize most of the literature on these subjects. We discuss use of these studies and others published within the past few decades to examine both the hypothesis that 'depression or the use of prescribed antidepressant medication causes cancer' and the association between cancer and the risk for major depression. We also describe the limited literature on culture and socioeconomic status in causing depression after a diagnosis of cancer.

THE CULTURAL CONTEXT

Culture can be defined as a system of values that may be reflected in the institutions, ethics, morals and political governance of a society. Ethnicity can be viewed as an expression of cultural belonging and is often defined as a common homeland (with a certain dominant cultural discourse) or a common language, although numerous definitions are used [3].

The cultural context of depression can be investigated both at the international level (by comparing its prevalence in countries with different dominating cultures) and at the national level (by comparing its prevalence amongst ethnic groups residing in the same country). Studies at both levels are important for disentangling the role of culture in depression. International studies have shown wide variation in the burden of depression, the percentage of total disability-adjusted life years lost being about 9% in high-income countries and about 4% in low-income countries [4]. An epidemiological study of the prevalence of depression in a number of European countries also showed wide variation by country and by urban and rural residence, rural areas having a higher prevalence [5]. Although the results at the international level support the hypothesis of cultural differences in depression, these differences may be due to other underlying factors, such as socioeconomic status (SES).

At the national level, mixed results have been obtained for an association between ethnicity and depression. One population-based study of immigrants to the Netherlands showed a higher overall level of depressive symptoms amongst Turkish and Moroccan immigrants than amongst native Dutch persons [6]. In the United States, a higher prevalence of depression was found amongst non-Hispanic whites than other groups [7]. These studies might, however, have been strongly influenced by the definition of the ethnic groups (e.g. first-generation immigrants or language preference) and by differences in SES in the new country and in the country of origin. Moreover, the patterns of depression by ethnicity at both national and international levels may be related to a number of other factors [8], including structural factors (differences in risk factors for depression such as stress and SES and differences in access to mental healthcare due perhaps to discrimination) and cultural factors (differences in the interpretation of feelings and symptoms, in recognition of depression as a disease, and in help-seeking behaviour and rules for expressing emotion). Also, languages have often been suggested to carry different propensities to represent mental distress, although a recent study found similar language and metaphors regarding somatization across ethnic groups [8].

The results of several studies support the hypothesis that depression can be influenced by differences in the interpretation of feelings and symptoms. A qualitative study in the United States of the conceptual model of depression showed that 36 South-Asian Americans mainly interpreted vignettes of depression in social and moral terms and considered that depression should be self-managed, while 37 European Americans mainly interpreted the vignettes in biological terms [9]. Another study showed cultural differences in the expression of depression: Chinese patients with depression had more somatic symptoms than European Canadians, who reported more psychological symptoms [10]. A study in an inner-city area in the United Kingdom with mixed methods, in which people of Pakistani origin were compared with whites did not, however, show a difference in somatization or in the prevalence of depressive disorders (12.3% vs. 9.0%) [8]. The hypothesis that differences in the prevalence of depression by ethnic group might be due to differences in the interpretation, recognition, or expression of depression is still controversial, and the role of structural factors, including SES and access to care, should not be underestimated [11].

SOCIAL DISPARITY

The relation between SES and health has been well established [12]. Studies of SES involve exploring what social and economic factors affect the positions that individuals and groups hold within a social structure [12]. The difficulty in disentangling the true effect of SES lies in the disparity between indicators, which are measurable, and the underlying constructs. Most epidemiological studies focus on indicators of 'life chances', such as education, occupation, employment status, income, affluence, pension, dwelling, geographical area, marital status, gender, or caste, as well as ethnic-based constructs, such as Afro-American in the United States and Aboriginal in Australia. Many European studies included measures of occupation, while those in the United States had measures of education and income [11]. Such measures are based on the assumption that it is the skills, knowledge and resources of an individual that link his/her position in the social structure with health. Indicators of SES may, however, be less closely linked to the individual and can include area-based measures, for instance of deprivation [11].

Studies of the influence of the political system on shaping inequalities in health have also been reported [13], and other studies have suggested a role of subjective SES [14]. A study of the process behind subjective SES suggested that individuals compare themselves with similar people, and that differences between objective and subjective SES are related to differences in perceived opportunities [15]. SES indicators can be used only as approximations of the characteristics for a given SES. It may be argued that SES itself is associated with disease, for instance, for indicators such as quality of dwelling (for example, access to clean water, sewer systems, air quality, or light), which may be a direct indicator of exposure to health-damaging factors. The position an individual holds within a social structure represents resources and limitations that are more indirectly important for health: for example, education may confer knowledge that initiates certain health behaviour.

SES can influence health through three general mechanisms [16]. Different SES is associated with different probabilities for health-damaging exposure; different probabilities of having health-protective resources to counteract exposure; and the effect of time in these exposure–resource combinations, as more negative exposure and fewer protective resources will take a toll on health over time, thus increasing susceptibility. The exposure–resource characteristics of the environments in which people live are thus 'embodied' over time [12, 17].

Studies of SES in relation to health often focus on disparities, which the World Health Organization has defined as 'differences in health which are not only unnecessary and avoidable but, in addition, are considered unfair and unjust' [18], suggesting that potential differences in health between advantaged and less advantaged groups may be systematic and potentially shaped by policies [19]. Examining disparities in health may be relevant for both low- and high-income countries and other settings where opportunities are not equal.

THE DANISH SETTING

Several studies of the effect of SES on health have been carried out in Denmark, for a number of reasons. Each Nordic country has a civil registration system, with unique personal identification numbers, national population-based administrative and health-related registries, and legislation that permits and supports registry-based research. In 1981, Denmark was the first country in the world to replace the questionnaire-based census usually conducted every five years by an annual register-based census. Danish society has a tax-paid welfare system, often referred to as 'the Scandinavian welfare model', which is characterized by free healthcare, free education, benefits for families with children and for people in the educational system, pensions and services for the elderly and disabled, and financial support for unemployed people. The Danish welfare model is subsidized by the state, and, as a result, Denmark has one of the highest taxation levels in the world, public expenditure accounting for 26% of the total gross domestic product. An exception is unemployment benefits, which are not covered by taxes alone but also through individual voluntary membership in unemployment funds, usually aligned with a given union.

Denmark has the largest workforce in Europe relative to its population. The high frequency of labour activity in Denmark is due in particular to the high proportion of women active in the labour market (approximately 70%); the respective proportion of men is

80%. Agreements within the Danish labour market make it highly flexible with regard to working hours, overtime and the hiring and firing of personnel. This also results in high mobility. In return for this high level of flexibility, Danish employees have relatively comprehensive social security, which is guaranteed by law in times of unemployment, illness, or occupational injury.

Denmark has a tax-funded healthcare system, which provides free access to general practice, outpatient and hospital care. The healthcare system is organized into a primary sector of general practitioners and specialists, who are under contract to or paid by the national health insurance, and a secondary sector, which operates hospitals under the authority of the national regions or the Danish state. General practitioners play a pivotal role as gatekeepers to the rest of the healthcare system, carrying out initial diagnostic investigations and making referrals to hospitals or outpatient clinics, as needed. Exceptions to free healthcare include dental care and prescription medications, which are only partly subsidized by the state. The conditions for carrying out population-based cancer research in Denmark and in the other Nordic countries are thus unique.

DOES DEPRESSION OR ANTIDEPRESSANT MEDICATION CAUSE CANCER?

Personality, mental vulnerability, and other factors related to the mind have long been considered in many societies to affect the risk for cancer. The idea that stress, major life events, personality traits, or depression cause cancer has not, however, been confirmed in studies with methods that address issues such as recall bias by the use of administrative information about the exposure under study, detailed, precise information about cancer morbidity and mortality, and the use of nationwide, population-based cancer registries.

We investigated the cancer risk of patients hospitalized for depression in a nationwide Danish cohort study. We combined information from two nationwide, population-based Danish registries to obtain complete data on depression, without selection bias. Information on hospitalization for affective disorders was obtained from the nationwide Danish Psychiatric Central Register, which, since 1969, has collected information on all admissions to psychiatric inpatient facilities, both psychiatric hospitals and psychiatric departments in general hospitals, and, since 1995, information from outpatient contacts [20]. All 89 491 adults in Denmark who had been admitted to a hospital with depression, as defined in the ICD-8, between 1969 and 1993 were identified, resulting in 1 117 006 person–years of follow-up through 1995. The incidence rates of all cancers and of site-specific cancers were compared with national incidence rates for first primary cancers, the analyses being adjusted for gender, age and calendar time. A total of 9922 cases of cancer were diagnosed in the cohort, with 9434.6 having been expected; this yielded a standardized incidence ratio of 1.05 (95% CI: 1.03–1.07). The risk for cancer was increased during the first year after hospital admission, with brain cancer occurring more frequently than expected, probably due to misclassification of depression. When the first year of follow-up was excluded, the increase was attributable mainly to increased risks for tobacco-related cancers: the standardized incidence ratios for non-tobacco-related cancers were 1.00 (95% CI, 0.97; 1.03) after 1–9 years of follow-up and 0.99 (95% CI: 0.95–1.02) after 10 or more years of follow-up. These results provide no support for the hypothesis that depression independently increases the risk for cancer, but they emphasize the deleterious effect that depression can have on lifestyle [21].

The study did not include information on depressive conditions that did not lead to hospital admission; however, we did study the risk for cancer amongst users of antidepressant medication, because an increased risk for non-Hodgkin lymphoma had been reported amongst long-term users of tricyclic antidepressants. The incidence amongst 43 932 users of any antidepressant medication (two or more prescriptions) in the county of North Jutland, Denmark, during 1989–2003 was compared with the incidence amongst all the remaining inhabitants of the county (about 500 000) who did not use antidepressants (one or no prescription). We used Poisson regression analysis and adjusted for age, gender, period and use of immunosuppressive drugs, corticosteroids, or nonsteroidal anti-inflammatory drugs. Use of tricyclic antidepressants was associated with an overall increased incidence of non-Hodgkin lymphoma (adjusted incidence rate ratio, 1.53; 95% CI: 1.06–2.21) when compared with non-use. The incidence rate ratio for users with 10 or more prescriptions and 5 or more years of follow-up was 2.50 (95% CI: 1.43–4.34). Our results indicated an increased risk for non-Hodgkin lymphoma specifically amongst long-term users of tricyclic antidepressants, and this finding is supported by an updated analysis showing that the increase in risk was confined to long-term heavy users of these antidepressants [22]. We did not observe increased risks for other cancers in users of more recently marketed antidepressants [23], indicating that, despite the association with use of tricyclic antidepressants, there is no convincing evidence that antidepressant medication causes cancer at any specific site.

SOCIAL DISPARITY, CANCER RISK AND SURVIVAL

Associations between indicators of SES and the incidence of different cancers are heterogeneous. For instance, low SES has been more or less consistently associated with increased risks for cancers of the cervix, head and neck, lung and stomach and lower risks for cancers of the breast, prostate and colon and malignant melanoma. Although the available information is sparse, longitudinal data suggest that differences in the risks for some types of cancers depending on SES are increasing [24]. These differences may be partly due to known risk factors, such as smoking, alcohol intake, occupational exposure, reproductive behaviour, and infectious agents (human papillomavirus, Helicobacter pylori, hepatitis B and C viruses), although few epidemiological studies have addressed this hypothesis directly.

We carried out a study of all 3.22 million Danish residents born between the years 1925 and 1973, who were followed up for cancer incidence in 1994–2003 and for survival in 1994–2006, yielding 147 973 cancers. Information on socioeconomic and demographic indicators for the study was obtained from the population-based Integrated Database for Labour Market Research in Statistics Denmark, which contains yearly data since 1980 [25]. For all persons in the study, we obtained information at the individual level on six socioeconomic indicators: education, disposable income, affiliation to the work market, social class, housing tenure, and size of dwelling. We also defined three demographic indicators: cohabitation status, type of district, and ethnicity. The incidence of cancer increased with lower education and income, especially for tobacco- and other lifestyle-related cancers. Social disparity in the prognosis of most cancers was observed, despite the equal access to healthcare in Denmark, with poorer relative survival related to fewer social advantages, and this social disparity was often most pronounced in the first year after diagnosis.

To varying degrees, differences in health in general, and in cancer in particular, by SES can be explained by differences in health behaviour. Several studies have indicated that poorer health behaviour is concentrated in less advantaged groups [26], and this might be exacerbated for behaviours like tobacco smoking [27], alcohol consumption, and physical inactivity, all of which have been associated with both the incidence of and survival from certain cancers.

A Danish study of population mortality, based on data from the Organization for Economic Co-operation and Development for 20 Western countries, showed that, in 1990–1999, the level of daily smoking amongst Danish men was the fourth highest (42%) and that amongst Danish women was the highest (36%). Alcohol use was the fifth highest of 15 Western countries, with an average consumption of 10.3 litres per person per year. The World Health Organization MONICA study, conducted in the first half of the 1990s, however, showed that Danes had some of the lowest levels of being overweight (41% of men and 26% of women) and obesity (13% of men and 12% of women) amongst the 10 Western European countries surveyed [28]. Thus, the observed disparity in cancer in Denmark is likely related to tobacco smoking and alcohol consumption.

SOCIAL DISPARITY AND DEPRESSION

Several studies have revealed associations between SES and depression [29, 30] and use of antidepressant medication [31]. We examined the distribution of SES in patients with depression amongst 3.4 million adult Danes. As shown in Table 9.1, more people with lower than higher income and education were hospitalized for an affective disorder. This finding was confirmed in a Danish study of 9254 people with registry-based information on SES factors, which showed a

Table 9.1 Hospitalization for depression by income and education amongst 3.4 million adult Danes

	N (%)	Ever hospitalized for depression (%)
Total population	3 403 004	4.7
Disposable income		
Low (1st quartile)	798 458 (23.5)	5.6
Medium (2nd–3rd quartile)	1 616 849 (47.5)	5.4
High (4th quartile)	819 931 (24.1)	2.3
None or unknown	167 766 (4.9)	6.1
Educational attainment		
Basic or high school	1 179 855 (34.7)	6.6
Vocational	1 241 867 (36.5)	3.8
Higher	895 221 (26.3)	3.5
Unknown	86 061 (2.6)	5.3

social gradient in depressive disorders, regardless of whether SES was measured as education, occupation, employment, or income [29].

Subjective social status has also been shown to be associated with depression [32]. Subjective measurement of SES may be especially relevant in studies of changes in SES in different ethnic groups, where the value for education may be unstable: for example, a degree from the country of origin might not be accepted in the new home country. A study of changes in subjective SES amongst Latino and Asian-American immigrants to the United States suggested that a subjective loss of SES was associated with increased risk for depressive episodes [33].

DEPRESSION AFTER A DIAGNOSIS OF CANCER

As more people survive cancer, it is important to understand its long-term impact. We therefore investigated whether cancer survivors are at increased risk for hospitalization for major depression. We linked data on all 5 703 754 persons living in Denmark on January 1, 1973, or born thereafter, to the Danish Cancer Registry and identified 608 591 adults with a diagnosis of cancer. We then followed these cancer patients for hospitalization for depression in the Danish Central Psychiatric Register from 1973 through 2003, which yielded 121 227 396 person-years and 121 304 hospitalizations for depression. The risk for depression in the first year after a cancer diagnosis was increased, with relative risks ranging from 1.16 (95% CI: 0.90–1.51) in women with colorectal cancer to 3.08 (95% CI: 1.88–5.02) in men with brain cancer. Decreasing, but still significant, excess risks were observed for most specific cancers during subsequent years. The risk remained increased throughout the study period for both men and women who survived hormone-related cancers, for women surviving smoking-related cancers, and for men surviving virus- and immune-related cancers. The study confirms that patients facing a life-threatening event like cancer are at increased risk for depression. This study probably shows only the tip of the iceberg, as we investigated the most severe forms of depression, that is, those requiring hospitalization [34].

CULTURAL DIFFERENCES IN DEPRESSION AFTER CANCER

To our knowledge, few studies have been performed on cultural differences in depression after a cancer diagnosis. In a recent Canadian study of 2402 people, an attempt was made to examine ethnic differences in distress after cancer. As it was found to be impossible to construct analytical groups by country or continent of origin, the authors examined differences between language groups (originating from a non-English- vs. an English-speaking country) and observed that people originating from non-English-speaking countries experienced more distress [35]. This suggests an association between ethnicity and depression, which could be related to structural factors, as language might be related to access to care.

SOCIAL DISPARITIES IN DEPRESSION AFTER CANCER AND THE IMPACT ON SURVIVAL

Few studies have examined whether the social disparity observed for depression is also seen for depression after a cancer diagnosis.

A Danish study of 3343 women with breast cancer showed that those who were economically disadvantaged had a higher prevalence of depressive symptoms than economically advantaged women [36]. A Chinese study of 1400 women with breast cancer also showed a higher prevalence amongst women with low income than those with high income [37]. Thus, there appears to be social disparity in depression after a cancer diagnosis in both high- and low-income countries.

The mechanisms behind social disparities in cancer survival include differences in stage at diagnosis, access to adequate and timely treatment as well as person-specific factors, like marital status and comorbidity by social group [38]. Depression is a disease that carries a high morbidity and mortality and has been found to be an independent prognostic factor amongst cancer patients in a number of epidemiological longitudinal studies (for example, [39–42]). Furthermore, depression has been associated with lesser adherence to cancer treatment regimen [43, 44].

Only very few studies have included depression as a possible prognostic factor in the analyses of social inequality in survival of cancer. The results of these few studies indicate that depression, due to a differential distribution by social class, might also contribute to the social gradient in prognosis after cancer [45, 46].

CONCLUSIONS

The importance of social disparities in health, and especially in cancer, has been clearly established, and the impact is striking. Indicators of SES, including health-damaging exposure, health-protective resources, and delay in seeking treatment, have been profoundly and consistently associated with a broad range of health and illness outcomes, in different countries and periods. Specific associations with different outcomes, such as suicide, heart disease, breast cancer, and depression, imply a social distribution of the relevant exposures and resources for these outcomes. One of the keys to understanding the heterogeneous strength and direction of the associations between markers of SES and certain outcomes is seeing how the social structure distributes risk and protective factors for a particular outcome to different SESs within that structure.

The role of culture in depression and in depression after cancer is complex. Some evidence suggests the involvement of cultural differences in the interpretation of feelings and symptoms of depression and in recognition of depression as a disorder. Still, many of the observed cultural differences in the prevalence of depression may be mediated through structural differences, including social disparity and disparity in access to care. The combined roles of culture and SES in causing depression after cancer should be further investigated in future epidemiological studies. Most studies on SES do not examine the mechanisms of and explanations for the role of SES and the health outcome; this is, however, essential, as SES is a multidimensional construct with numerous definitions and interpretations. We need further understanding of the overlap between culture and SES in depression after cancer and of the theoretical framework in which measures of SES are embedded, with the SES constructs behind measures of, for instance, income and education and the constructs of ethnicity and culture.

In this chapter, we have illustrated how the individual's risk for cancer, survival after cancer, and depression after cancer is influenced by his/her SES and, perhaps, by his/her ethnicity and culture, at both the international level in comparisons of countries and the national level in comparisons of group differences within a society. In countries with equal access to healthcare, such as Denmark, there should be no disparity in health outcomes, but there is.

Some of the main points raised in this chapter have been based on Danish population-based studies, and one could argue that some of the findings reported in those studies are likely to be specific to Danish circumstances, but we think that most of the findings we highlight are to some degree generalizable. Social inequality in health outcomes is an almost universal finding and so is the social gradient in cancer outcomes and in depression. Of course, the gradient may vary according to the population studied as may the relative importance of different mechanisms that mediate the gradients, but the findings we have summarized are relevant for all societies in which health interventions are established in accordance with the political goal of equal access to public health services.

How should health professionals deal with such disparity? It is time to challenge the paradigm in which we strive for equal access to healthcare and instead strive for equality in health outcome, which implies unequal access to care. This could be done by taking into account, in the healthcare system, SES characteristics such as income and education, social factors such as marital status, and health factors such as comorbidity and lifestyle. People with few resources and many health-damaging exposures should be offered a more comprehensive protocol of care. Changing the healthcare paradigm in this way will require political support to sustain everyday clinical work.

REFERENCES

1. Kendler, K.S., Gardner, C.O. and Prescott, C.A. (2002) Toward a comprehensive developmental model for major depression in women. *Am. J. Psychiatry*, **159**, 1133–1145.
2. Kendler, K.S., Gardner, C.O. and Prescott, C.A. (2006) Toward a comprehensive developmental model for major depression in men. *Am. J. Psychiatry*, **163**, 115–124.
3. Bauman, G. (1996) *Contesting Culture: Discourses of Identity in Multi-Ethnic*, Cambridge University Press, London, United Kingdom.
4. Ustun, T.B., Ayuso-Mateos, J.L., Chatterji, S. *et al.* (2004) Global burden of depressive disorders in the year 2000. *Br. J. Psychiatry*, **184**, 386–392.
5. Ayuso-Mateos, J.L., Vazquez-Barquero, J.L., Dowrick, C. *et al.* (2001) Depressive disorders in Europe: prevalence figures from the ODIN study. *Br. J. Psychiatry*, **179**, 308–316.
6. Schrier, A.C., de Wit, M.A., Rijmen, F., *et al.* Similarity in depressive symptom profile in a population-based study of migrants in the Netherlands. *Soc. Psychiatry Psychiatr. Epidemiol.* [Epub ahead of print].
7. Ohayon, M.M. (2007) Epidemiology of depression and its treatment in the general population. *J. Psychiatr. Res.*, **41**, 207–213.
8. Mallinson, S. and Popay, J. (2007) Describing depression: ethnicity and the use of somatic imagery in accounts of mental distress. *Sociol. Health Illn.*, **29**, 857–871.
9. Karasz, A. (2005) Cultural differences in conceptual models of depression. *Soc. Sci. Med.*, **60**, 1625–1635.
10. Ryder, A.G., Yang, J., Zhu, X. *et al.* (2008) The cultural shaping of depression: somatic symptoms in China, psychological symptoms in North America? *J. Abnorm. Psychol.*, **117**, 300–313.
11. Braveman, P.A., Cubbin, C., Egerter, S. *et al.* (2005) Socioeconomic status in health research: one size does not fit all. *JAMA*, **294**, 2879–2888.

12. Lynch, J. and Kaplan, G. (2000) Socioeconomic position, in *Social Epidemiology* (eds. L.F. Berkman and I. Kawachi), Oxford University Press, New York, pp. 13–35.

13. Beckfield, J. and Krieger, N. (2009) Epi + demos + cracy: linking political systems and priorities to the magnitude of health inequities–evidence, gaps, and a research agenda. *Epidemiol. Rev.*, **31**, 152–177.

14. Singh-Manoux, A., Adler, N.E. and Marmot, M.G. (2003) Subjective social status: its determinants and its association with measures of ill-health in the Whitehall II study. *Soc. Sci. Med.*, **56**, 1321–1333.

15. Franzini, L. and Fernandez-Esquer, M.E. (2006) The association of subjective social status and health in low-income Mexican-origin individuals in Texas. *Soc. Sci. Med.*, **63**, 788–804.

16. Davey Smith, G., Ben-Shlomo, Y. and Lynch, J. (2002) Lifecourse approaches to inequalities in coronary heart disease risk, in *Stress and the Heart: Psychosocial Pathways to Coronary Heart Disease* (eds. S. Stansfeld and M. Marmot), British Medical Journal Books, London, pp. 20–49.

17. Davey Smith, G., Gunnell, D. and Ben-Shlomo, Y. (2001) Lifecourse approaches to socio-economic differentials in cause-specific adult mortality, in *Power, Inequality and Health* (eds. D. Leon and G. Walt), Oxford University Press, Oxford.

18. Whitehead, M. (1992) The concepts and principles of equity and health. *Int. J. Health Serv.*, **22**, 429–445.

19. James, S.A. (2009) Epidemiologic research on health disparities: some thoughts on history and current developments. *Epidemiol. Rev.*, **31**, 1–6.

20. Munk-Jorgensen, P. and Mortensen, P.B. (1997) The Danish Psychiatric Central Register. *Dan. Med. Bull.*, **44**, 82–84.

21. Dalton, S.O., Mellemkjaer, L., Olsen, J.H. *et al.* (2002) Depression and cancer risk: a register-based study of patients hospitalized with affective disorders, Denmark, 1969-1993. *Am. J. Epidemiol.*, **155**, 1088–1095.

22. Dalton, S.O., Poulsen, A.H., Norgaard, M. *et al.* (2008) Tricyclic antidepressants and non-Hodgkin lymphoma. *Epidemiology*, **19**, 546–549.

23. Dalton, S.O., Johansen, C., Mellemkjaer, L. *et al.* (2000) Antidepressant medications and risk for cancer. *Epidemiology*, **11**, 171–176.

24. Faggiano, F., Partane, T., Kogevinas, M. and Boffeta, P. (1997) Socio-economic differences in cancer incidence and mortality, in *Social Inequalities and Cancer* (eds. M. Kogevinas, N. Pearce, M. Susser and P. Boffetta), International Agency for Research on Cancer, Lyon, pp. 65–176.

25. Thygesen, L. (1995) The register-based system of demographic and social statistics in Denmark. *Stat. J. UN Econ. Comm. Eur.*, **12**, 49–55.

26. Groth, M.V., Fagt, S., Stockmarr, A. *et al.* (2009) Dimensions of socioeconomic position related to body mass index and obesity among Danish women and men. *Scand. J. Public Health*, **37**, 418–426.

27. Statens Institut for Folkesundhed (2005) *Langt færre rygere blandt højt uddannede end blandt lavt uddannede*, Statens Institut for Folke-sundhed, Copenhagen.

28. Juel, K. (2004) *Dødeligheden I. Danmark gennem 100 å. Danskerne lever længere men hvorfor 3-4 å kortere end svenske mænd og franske kvinder*, National Danish Institute of Public Health, Copenhagen.

29. Andersen, I., Thielen, K., Nygaard, E. and Diderichsen, F. (2009) Social inequality in the prevalence of depressive disorders. *J. Epidemiol. Community Health*, **63**, 575–581.

30. Stansfeld, S.A., Head, J., Fuhrer, R. *et al.* (2003) Social inequalities in depressive symptoms and physical functioning in the Whitehall II study: exploring a common cause explanation. *J. Epidemiol. Community Health*, **57**, 361–367.

31. Hansen, D.G., Sondergaard, J., Vach, W. *et al.* (2004) Socio-economic inequalities in first-time use of antidepressants: a population-based study. *Eur. J. Clin. Pharmacol.*, **60**, 51–55.

32. Demakakos, P., Nazroo, J., Breeze, E. and Marmot, M. (2008) Socio-economic status and health: the role of subjective social status. *Soc. Sci. Med.*, **67**, 330–340.

33. Nicklett, E.J. and Burgard, S.A. (2009) Downward social mobility and major depressive episodes among Latino and Asian-American immi-grants to the United States. *Am. J. Epidemiol.*, **170**, 793–801.

34. Dalton, S.O., Laursen, T.M., Ross, L. *et al.* (2009) Risk for hospitaliza-tion with depression after a cancer diagnosis: a nationwide, population-based study of cancer patients in Denmark from 1973 to 2003. *J. Clin. Oncol.*, **27**, 1440–1445.

35. Thomas, B.C., Carlson, L.E. and Bultz, B.D. (2009) Cancer patient ethnicity and associations with emotional distress – the 6th vital sign: a new look at defining patient ethnicity in a multicultural context. *J. Immigr. Minor Health*, **11**, 237–248.

36. Christensen, S., Zachariae, R., Jensen, A.B. *et al.* (2009) Prevalence and risk of depressive symptoms 3-4 months post-surgery in a nationwide cohort study of Danish women treated for early stage breast-cancer. *Breast Cancer Res. Treat.*, **113**, 339–355.

37. Chen, X., Zheng, Y., Zheng, W. *et al.* (2009) Prevalence of depression and its related factors among Chinese women with breast cancer. *Acta Oncol.*, **48**, 1128–1136.

38. Woods, L.M., Rachet, B. and Coleman, M.P. (2006) Origins of socio-economic inequalities in cancer survival: a review. *Ann. Oncol.*, **17**, 5–19.

39. Watson, M., Haviland, J.S., Greer, S. *et al.* (1999) Influence of psychological response on survival in breast cancer: a population-based cohort study. *Lancet*, **354**, 1331–1336.

40. Brown, K.W., Levy, A.R., Rosberger, Z. and Edgar, L. (2003) Psychological distress and cancer survival: a follow-up 10 years after diagnosis. *Psychosom. Med.*, **65**, 636–643.

41. Faller, H. and Schmidt, M. (2004) Prognostic value of depressive coping and depression in survival of lung cancer patients. *Psychooncology*, **13**, 359–363.

42. Prieto, J.M., Atala, J., Blanch, J. *et al.* (2005) Role of depression as a predictor of mortality among cancer patients after stem-cell transplantation. *J. Clin. Oncol.*, **23**, 6063–6071.

43. Fann, J.R., Thomas-Rich, A.M., Katon, W.J. *et al.* (2008) Major depression after breast cancer: a review of epidemiology and treatment. *Gen. Hosp. Psychiatry*, **30**, 112–126.

44. Kissane, D.W. (2009) Beyond the psychotherapy and survival debate: the challenge of social disparity, depression and treatment adherence in psychosocial cancer care. *Psychooncology*, **18**, 1–5.

45. Frederiksen, B.L., Osler, M., Harling, H. *et al.* (2009) Do patient characteristics, disease, or treatment explain social inequality in survival from colorectal cancer? *Soc. Sci. Med.*, **69**, 1107–1115.

46. Dalton, S.O., Ross, L., During, M. *et al.* (2007) Influence of socioeconomic factors on survival after breast cancer – a nationwide cohort study of women diagnosed with breast cancer in Denmark 1983-1999. *Int. J. Cancer*, **121**, 2524–2531.

Acknowledgement

The World Psychiatric Association gratefully acknowledges the support of the following donors for this initiative: the Lugli Foundation in Rome, the Italian Society of Biological Psychiatry, Eli Lilly and Bristol-Myers Squibb.

Index

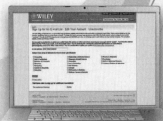